"The American Cancer Society is deeply indebted to Judi Johnson and Pat Norby for developing the I CAN COPE program, which has helped so many cancer patients and their families. This companion resource book expands on that program and provides extensive useful information."

> Harmon J. Eyre, M.D.
> Deputy Executive Vice President for Medical Affairs and Research
> American Cancer Society, Atlanta, Georgia

"This is a comprehensive resource for cancer patients and their families to use throughout their treatment and follow-up care."

> J. Paul Van Nevel
> Associate Director for Cancer Communications
> National Cancer Institute, Bethesda, Maryland

"When you learn you have cancer, you don't want to go it alone. You need competent medical care, good information, and a supportive environment of family and friends. In a straightforward and hopeful manner, I CAN COPE provides guidance in all these areas. This book teaches the person with cancer how to be a team player and end up a winner."

> Harvey Mackay, author of
> *Swim With the Sharks Without Being Eaten Alive*

"I CAN COPE is absolutely packed with highly readable information about all aspects of cancer. It is easily the most useful work of its kind I have seen and surely will prove of great value to cancer patients and their families, as well as their medical care providers."

> Irving J. Lerner, M.D., Oncologist
> 1992-93 President, Minnesota Society of Clinical Oncology,
> Minneapolis, Minnesota

". . . Straightforward, factual, and syr those concerned about cancer."

> *Library Journal*

GW00632259

"I CAN COPE should be mandatory reading for every cancer patient, friend, and relative, as well as every health care professional. It not only gives insight into the feelings, problems, and obstacles that will be encountered on the journey of the cancer patient, but also provides solid recommendations on how to meet and overcome these obstacles. This book has my highest recommendation."

> Richard A. Bloch
> Co-founder of H & R Block, lung cancer survivor, author and member of the National Cancer Advisory Board

"I found myself intrigued by each character in I CAN COPE. Their willingness to share concerns, pain, and hopes was mindful of ALL the students who have attended the I Can Cope course since it was developed over a decade ago. I CAN COPE is an exciting, realistic, and positive resource book that will benefit not only patients, but any person or health team member involved in the cancer issue."

> Pat Norby, R.N., O.C.N.
> Co-Founder of I CAN COPE

"This book has a positive message. It is about caring, about loving, about living life—not just facing it. It is a book that should be read by anyone who has been touched by cancer as a patient, relative, or friend."

> Harry Linduff
> Executive Vice President , American Cancer Society
> Minnesota Division

"A gem of a handbook."

> *Chicago Medicine*

I Can Cope

Staying Healthy with Cancer

by

Judi Johnson
&
Linda Klein

I Can Cope: Staying Healthy With Cancer—Revised and Updated
©1994 by Judi Johnson and Linda Klein.

Library of Congress Cataloging-in-Publication Data

Johnson, Judi, 1951-
I Can Cope: Staying Healthy With Cancer
Judi Johnson and Linda Klein.--Revised and updated 2nd edition.
        p.   cm.
Includes bibliographical references and index.
ISBN 1-56561-039-3   : $12.95
    1. Cancer--Patients--Rehabilitation
    2. Cancer--Psychological aspects.
    3.Adjustment (Psychology)
I. Klein, Linda, 1947-   II. Title.
RC262.J64   1994
616.99'4'0019--dc20   93-23399
                                        CIP

Cover Design: Emerson, Wajdowicz Studios, Inc./NYC
Interior Design: Liana Vaiciulis Raudys
Editor: Caroline Danielson

Published by
CHRONIMED Publishing
P.O. Box 47945
Minneapolis, MN 55447-9727

TABLE OF CONTENTS

Acknowledgements

Heartfelt thanks to—

All the people with cancer who shared intimate details of their personal lives and inspired us with their courage, determination, and positive views on life after cancer. Their collective wisdom and insight make up much of this book.

All the professional staff at North Memorial Medical Center, HealthEast St. Joseph's Hospital, and Lakeview Memorial Hospital for including us in their I CAN COPE classes and allowing us to tape material for use in this book.

Special people include—

Pat Norby, co-founder of I CAN COPE. Pat worked long hours to help steer the program from a dream to a reality.

Sister Ann Michelle Jadlowski and Sue Harvieux, who suggested some of the personalities we have highlighted. As I CAN COPE facilitators, both women have provided tremendous support to hundreds of cancer patients.

Dr. Irving Lerner, who willingly provided information, inspiration, and volunteer editing assistance to assure medical accuracy of the manuscript.

Harry Linduff and Betty Merriman at the National Office of the American Cancer Society who facilitated the collaboration of the newly revised patient education materials with the second edition of the book.

Our families and friends—Our husbands, Bill and Randy, tolerated hours of telephone conversations. Mary, Andrew, and Alison wondered why Mom was always at the computer. And several special friends encouraged and guided us toward completing this product. Thanks to all of you.

Foreword

A diagnosis of cancer significantly disrupts the lives of the affected patients and their families. The resources, information, and guidance provided by the American Cancer Society (ACS) can be a source of great relief for these people. This help comes in the form of counseling, patient education, support groups, visitation, home care, and patient transportation, just to name a few.

Meeting the needs of cancer patients and their families on a local level has always been a priority of the Society. The I CAN COPE program specifically combines education with the skills and coping tools needed by these people. For this reason, in 1977, the Minnesota Division welcomed Judi Johnson's proposal to develop a patient education program to address this issue and provide these services. The goal of this program is empowerment through education. The Minnesota Division program was a significant success—so m___ ___ it was considered a model program and was adopted _____ n Cancer Society. How many patie___ ___ is program? Undoubtedly, hundreds _____.

As the second edition of this b__ ___ I CAN COPE program is being in_____ ry. While Judi Johnson and Linda ____ ___ his book, they have been involve__ ___ the revised program as well. As ___ for Division Services at the Soci___ e in Atlanta, I see remarkable evi___ the I CAN COPE program has becor__ it is the volunteers with their exp___ and commitment to patient servic___ ss.

This book provides the co___ I CAN COPE program. But it is only a one-dim_____ ng of a

ix

three-dimensional concept. Attending I CAN COPE classes, working with health care professionals from your area, and meeting
other people with cancer deepens and broadens the message and
brings it home to the heart. I hope the reading of this book will
serve as a catalyst and inspire people to pick up the phone and
call their local ACS unit or division office to find the time and
place of the next I CAN COPE class in their area. Bring the book
along. Use it as a reference. Experience the benefits of I CAN
COPE first hand in the supportive environment of your local
community.

Harry Linduff, Group Vice President
Division Wide Services
American Cancer Society
National Office, Atlanta, Georgia

Introduction

This is a book about differences. It is about the difference between dying of cancer and learning to live with cancer. It is about the difference between people who say "I'm afraid to die" and people who say "I want to live." It is about the difference between allowing cancer to control you and gaining control of your cancer. It is about being healthy despite a cancer diagnosis.

Bill's testicular cancer was first diagnosed when he was 26 years old. He underwent surgery and one year of chemotherapy, which put the cancer into remission. Ten years later, a sophisticated blood test told doctors Bill's cancer was back. More chemotherapy, then more surgery followed. And today Bill is cancer free again.

When Malinda had breast cancer surgery, doctors discovered a rare inflammatory type of cancer which had already spread to more than 20 of her lymph nodes. She immediately started chemotherapy and enjoyed a short-term remission. But within a year the cancer had spread to her bones. She began an aggressive treatment program that included two weeks of continuous chemotherapy every month.

Yet both of these people consider themselves healthy. Cancer and healthy. Are the words compatible? Bill and Malinda think so, and so do we.

We know that people with cancer and their families can learn to adjust to a cancer diagnosis and continue to live healthy lives. They have proven that time and again. But to do that, they need help. And that's why I CAN COPE came into being.

In my work as an oncology nurse, I started thinking about developing a patient education program that would serve the needs of these people. I mentioned my idea to Pat Norby, another oncology nurse. She agreed wholeheartedly that we were watching patients leave the hospital unprepared to deal with the physical and emotional impact of their newly diagnosed illness. These people were alone and afraid. They didn't know anyone with cancer. They didn't know anything about cancer.

To serve those needs, the I CAN COPE program was born. Pat and I broke the educational package into eight sessions, and we had two goals in mind. First, we wanted to help people find a balance between fatalistically accepting their disease and unrealistically resisting it. Second, through education and support from others, we believed people with cancer could begin to regain control of their lives.

I CAN COPE was first presented as a research project at North Memorial Medical Center in Minneapolis. It gained the support of the Minnesota Division of the American Cancer Society, and today it is one of the American Cancer Society's service and rehabilitation programs. The course is offered in almost every state throughout the United States.

For thousands of people across the country, I CAN COPE has made the difference between coping and giving up. By offering an educational program in a supportive environment, the I CAN COPE program has helped these people make conscious decisions to accept their disease and learn to live with it. It steered them toward a balanced life after a most unbalancing event–the cancer diagnosis.

Almost every aspect of life changes after the diagnosis. I CAN COPE was designed to help people go through those changes with the least amount of trauma. But what about all the people who are unable or unwilling to participate in I CAN COPE classes? When Linda Klein came to me with the idea of writing a book about the I CAN COPE program, I knew that would be the vehicle that could take the message out of the classroom and into people's homes. After interviewing many class participants, we chose to follow several of them and teach the lessons of I CAN COPE through their eyes.

These are ordinary people, but when cancer became a part of their lives, they became extraordinary people. Their stories are both heart-wrenching and uplifting. They are filled with both pain and courage. They are stories of people struggling to achieve that delicate balance between accepting cancer without resistance—and resisting cancer without acceptance.

All of these people had to learn a new way of achieving balance in their lives. They couldn't simply give up on life. And yet they couldn't swing the other way and pretend their cancer didn't exist. Our book offers suggestions to help people stabilize their lives and regain a sense of balance.

For those who are denying and refusing to accept the cancer diagnosis, it is important to take concrete steps toward facing reality:

- Learn to say the word cancer.
- Learn about options available to you.
- Acknowledge the possible outcomes.

People who are accepting cancer as their fate and refusing to fight back need to become more involved in living:

- Be totally honest with yourself and others by learning to complain and share your concerns.
- Guard against depression by setting concrete goals for the future and blocking out negative thoughts.
- Refuse to be limited, either by yourself or your health care team.

Since being diagnosed with breast cancer, Malinda has learned the meaning of balance. "There are three kinds of cancer patients," she says. "First is the person who lies back and says, 'I'm going to die.' That person probably will die. Another person may deny the existence of cancer and refuse to accept help. Then there is the third kind, the kind I've tried to be. I cooperate with my doctor and trust his judgment. But in the end, I am responsible for my own health. I have tried to work that way since I was first diagnosed and through many difficult times."

And there will be difficult times. But we hope that reading this book and sharing the intimate experiences of several people who have attended the eight sessions of I CAN COPE will enable people to adapt the same coping skills to their own lives. Our goal is to help people put cancer in its place so they can get on with living.

Today, more people are living with cancer than ever before. Nearly 50 percent of all people diagnosed with cancer this year can expect to be cured. For those who will not be cured, new methods of treatment are now extending life and, in many cases, also enhancing its quality.

You make the difference. You can make the choice between dying of cancer and learning to live with cancer. We believe our book will help you achieve the balance necessary to take control and live a healthy life.

Judi Johnson, R.N., Ph.D., FAAN

This Book Is Dedicated To:

Bill
Dave
Debbie
Dick
Hazel
Jim
John
Lothair
Lou
Malinda

with whom it has been an honor
and a privilege to work.

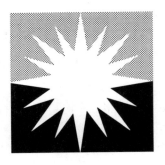

"My mind swings from

disbelief to fatalism. I am

vacillating between a

surging belief that all will be

well and a maudlin conviction

that nothing will ever be

right again."

Cornelius Ryan
A Private Battle

The Diagnosis

You have cancer.

With those three words, the lives of the people in this chapter were instantly changed. To hear the words was devastating. To pick up the pieces and go forward seemed impossible at the time. And for them, the roller coaster ride had just begun.

The Stories

Dave

Dave and Loretta think back to before "all this happened" and describe a wonderful life. Both had successful careers, complete with master's degrees in their individual fields. Their two grown daughters had never rebelled and tested their parents to the limit. As a family, they played together, prayed together, and stayed together. They owned a comfortable home in a quiet suburb, surrounded by mature trees and just enough nature to make the setting seem rural rather than urban. They had developed a network of good friends. Loretta summed it up well when she commented, "I would say we had an ideal life." Ideal until Dave's diagnosis of Hodgkin's disease threw them into a tailspin.

The spin was actually a slow spiral from control to loss of control, since Dave's diagnosis didn't come with the rapid-fire certainty one might hope for. Up to age 50, Dave felt great. Then he developed symptoms suggesting rheumatoid arthritis and his health started to deteriorate. "I was working out daily and feeling good about my physical condition," he remembers. All of a sudden his joints started swelling. Knees. Elbows. Fingers. To the point where he could no longer exercise. For the next year, a rheumatologist treated Dave's arthritis with various medications, including gold and prednisone.

1

In the meantime, other symptoms started to surface, beginning with night sweats. At first Dave suspected a leak in their waterbed. They eventually discovered a pinhole in the mattress, but it was on Loretta's side of the bed. Dave's nocturnal drenching worsened, with no apparent external cause. They joked about it, Loretta accusing Dave of going through "manopause." As time went on, Dave found himself changing pajamas two or three times a night. When he ran a fever of 105 degrees, they panicked and called a doctor, who soothed them and convinced them not to worry.

Then the aches started, first in Dave's abdomen. "If I had a drink on Friday night, I felt like someone had put a fist in my stomach." Soon the aches spread throughout his body, most noticeably in his back. But that didn't stop Dave from continuing his full-time selling job and traveling all week at times. He just packed three heating pads to allay the body aches and keep him comfortable.

By this time, Dave's rheumatologist had taken him off all medications. Dave wonders now if the doctor suspected something more serious and just didn't say anything. Finally the dramatic vacillation between chills and high fevers couldn't be ignored any longer. "I came out of a meeting with an episode of chills on an unusually warm April day. It was 90 degrees outside, I had the heat on full blast in my car, and I couldn't get warm." Once the chills subsided, his temperature spiked immediately.

He was referred to a gastroenterologist. After several uncomfortable tests (including barium and endoscopic studies), the doctor suggested Dave needed to have his gallbladder removed. "I said no," Loretta interjects emphatically. "My nursing background told me he was not a candidate for gallbladder surgery." She enlisted the help of a trusted friend and surgeon. He zeroed in on Dave's symptoms almost immediately. The surgeon removed a small lymph node from under Dave's arm, looked at the cells, and did a bone marrow biopsy. The results revealed a Stage IV Hodgkin's disease.

"I still have a lot of guilt that I didn't recognize what was going on," Loretta says. In retrospect, she would have expected to see some swelling in his neck. As it turned out, swollen lymph nodes proved to be the one missing symptom on Dave's long road to diagnosis, a journey that lasted 18 months before his cancer was confirmed.

Dick

When Dick learned he had lung cancer, it was the first time he had come face to face with death. Today, wispy hairs flying in all directions off a nearly bald head are the only visible reminder of the disease that "scared the hell" out of him.

"I used to have a pretty good head of hair," Dick admits ruefully. "Now I hardly get my money's worth when I go for a haircut." Dick received 10 radiation treatments to his brain after surgery to remove two cancerous lobes from his right lung. Most people get all their hair back after undergoing chemotherapy. But that is not the case with radiation.

"If I had to do it over again, I might not go through with the radiation. On the other hand, if I had a choice between talking to you today and my hair. . . ." His voice trails off, but the decision he would make is obvious.

At 45, Dick had been a ripe candidate for lung cancer. His grandmother died of breast cancer, and his father died of lymphoma when he was 45. In addition, Dick picked up his first cigarette when he was 14, and except for three years in his mid-thirties, he smoked two packs a day until age 44. What made him quit then? Listening to his brother coughing during a family reunion.

Dick went to California for a long-overdue reunion with his three brothers. Separated since the death of their parents, the boys had hardly seen one another for years. It was then that Dick realized all the brothers had one bad habit in common: smoking. "My one brother smokes Camels," Dick recalls. "No filters. To hear him get started in the morning would be comical if it weren't so tragic. His coughing sounds like a diesel truck trying to start." Dick knew he didn't sound much better. When he returned home, he made an appointment with a quit-smoking clinic for the first week after Labor Day. "It cost me $400, but I quit."

The following August, Dick developed what he thought was a summer cold. But after listening to him cough and hack for more than three weeks, several of his seven children started nagging him about going to the doctor. In addition, one of his co-workers at the graphic arts shop was also after him.

Dick gave in and saw a doctor. The diagnosis was bronchitis, and Dick went home with two weeks' worth of antibiotics. But when that didn't work, the doctors took a chest X-ray and compared it to one taken one year earlier. The new picture showed a spot on the right lung. The doctor immediately sent Dick to a lung specialist.

The specialist ran several tests, all with inconclusive results. He decided surgery was in order. "He told me before the operation that it could be a virus, tuberculosis, or cancer," Dick said. "He thought there was about a 30 percent chance it could be cancer."

Dick was scheduled for surgery in October. Because the lung specialist had downplayed the possibility it could be cancer, Dick was not overly concerned about the surgery. He recalls that "the one thing that really worried me was if and when I would be able to use my arm again." The operation was on his right side. The surgeon had explained that he would be cutting arm muscles, lifting the shoulder blade, and taking a rib out. Dick remembers cautioning the doctor. "I told him be careful. If I can't use my arm, I can't make a living."

Dick was alone in his room watching a football game when the lung specialist came in to give him the results of the surgery. "He didn't even turn off the TV to talk to me," Dick remembers uneasily. The spot was cancer, and the surgeon had removed two of the three lobes of his right lung.

Dick believes that "for the average person, which I consider myself, finding out you have cancer is like a death sentence. He couldn't have done more to me if he had looked me in the eye and said, 'You're going to die.' Starting at the bottom like that, I knew it would be uphill from there."

Debbie

For most of her life, tall, willowy Debbie had been fighting one battle after another. Now, at 26, she was faced with a malignant brain tumor that was threatening to cut that life short. "Sure, I was angry," she confesses. "But what can you do? It's there, and you can't fight it. I've fought many battles, but this is one thing I can't do anything about."

Debbie tugs self-consciously at what is left of her once-thick blond hair. She talks about being the oldest of three children. After spending eight years as an only child, Debbie encountered her first battle—adjusting to the birth of her baby sister. As she recalls, "My mom says I hated my sister because I wasn't the only child anymore. I said I didn't. But maybe I did. She was a perfect baby, where I had been a terror. My mom and dad nicknamed her Happy Time." But it wasn't a happy time for Debbie.

The ensuing years at home continued to be tense. Communication among family members was minimal. "It's not like we hated each other," she says. "It was more like five people living in the same house, but not together."

Although she and her mom fought about everything from boys to clothes, it was her dad Debbie really feared. She says he seldom spoke, and she never knew when he was going to get angry. He slept on the family couch. They called him Dad, but nobody really knew him. Strained relations between Debbie and her dad have been painful. But she says she would die before admitting it to him. "I know he has feelings inside, but he's like a brick wall. If you could get through the wall, I think he'd be a great person underneath."

Debbie was acutely aware of the rift between her and her parents even after leaving home. She says, "If I didn't make the effort to keep calling my family, I wouldn't know I had one."

Her real battle began while she was working for a cosmetics company in Houston, Texas. It was the first time she experienced what she terms "zoning out." "I would just stop, and for a split second I'd lose consciousness, although at the time I didn't realize what was happening. I could hear people and understand, but I couldn't answer back." It first occurred on a day when a bottle of pungent hair care solution had broken in the back room. She blamed it on the chemicals. While in Texas, Debbie continued having the attacks once every couple of months. She still thought it was caused by the environment.

But when she returned to Minnesota, the attacks didn't stop. "Then I thought it was just my body telling me to slow down because I'm a very hyper, fast-paced person." In addition, Debbie has a history of headaches, so head problems weren't new to her. But when one particular headache lasted six days, she became concerned. "It was different from the other ones," she remembers. "I can't explain how, but it just nagged me more."

She went to the local clinic, where the doctor asked her if she was having personal problems or was under a lot of stress. "I just laughed and told him my whole life has been stressful." He told her to take some time off and sent her home with a prescription for Valium (a tranquilizer) and Motrin (an anti-inflammatory medication) to break the chain of pain. She took some time off, took the pills, and the headache went away.

The headache was gone, but the attacks continued. A year later, they were becoming more frequent and lasting longer. Her friends were starting to notice. During an attack, Debbie would stop, make a face, and her lip would curl up. The attacks would usually last 15 or 20 seconds.

As soon as she was covered by insurance through her work, Debbie saw a neurologist. He ran several tests and determined she was healthy physically but perhaps had emotional problems. Her first EEG showed some abnormal brain waves, but the doctor said that was not unusual considering her history of headaches. They asked her to come back for another EEG and a CT (computerized tomography) scan of her head.

Early in July, Debbie stayed up all night and went in the next morning for a sleep-deprived EEG and CT scan. When she got home that afternoon, she received a phone call from one of the nurses in the CT room. They wanted more pictures. Right after that, her doctor called. He said they had found a spot and he wanted her back in the office the next day. He didn't want her to come alone.

"I thought, oh God, a spot and he doesn't want me to come in alone," Debbie exclaims. "This is just like the movies. I literally fell apart on the phone. I hadn't had any sleep in 24 hours, and now this." Although her mother was the first person she called, Debbie asked her boyfriend to go with her to hear the test results. She feared how her parents might react to bad news.

The next day, she went in for more X-rays. When the doctor called them into his office, reality hit home. "He hung that picture of my head up, and there was this dark blob. It was a spot all right. He had me thinking it was something so minute you couldn't see it. It was about a quarter of the size of my head."

Debbie's neurologist prepared her for the upcoming surgery with optimistic words of encouragement. He believed the tumor had been there a long time and would probably be classified as a Grade 1 or 2 tumor. There was a good chance it wouldn't be cancerous.

But it was cancer. And even after the spot was diagnosed as a Grade 3 malignant brain tumor, Debbie continued to receive mixed messages from her neurosurgeon. "My surgeon said he doesn't like to call it cancer," Debbie says. "He just said it was a form of cancer. I guess I was convinced that it wasn't serious and they had gotten it all. At that point, I felt lucky."

Jim

When Jim notice blood in his stool, both he and the doctors were convinced he had an ulcer. And he did. The only problem was that the ulcer was located on a softball-sized malignant tumor on the back of Jim's stomach.

After working 36 years as a designer for Northern States Power Company in Minneapolis, this new development had not been a part of Jim's master plan. At 58, he felt good and had expected to take early retirement. He and his wife Shirley enjoyed camping and planned to take their new camper around the country. Their three grown children and three grandchildren lived nearby, and Jim was hoping he would now have more time to spend with them.

Tall and square jawed, Jim's handsome face and quiet voice bring back memories of John Wayne. Shirley describes him as Mr. Cool—on the outside. According to her, "He never gets excited about anything. Always keeps an even temper. He never raises his voice. He is very calm, cool, and collected."

Jim admits that Shirley's description isn't exactly the truth. Although he maintained a cool exterior, life's pressures had a way of getting to him. "Bad news really bothered me. There were times when I felt depressed. Especially disappointments in not getting different jobs. I took them pretty hard. I don't think I ever really got rid of that stress. I kept most of it inside. Maybe if I had yelled and hollered a little bit, I would have been better off."

Jim admits he is a workaholic around the house. A neatly kept yard and freshly painted house and garage provide evidence of the time he devotes at home. Shirley concurs with that description. She describes him as "the kind of person who would get home from a three-week vacation, get everything unpacked, and then not be able to sit down until he had washed the car. He is a hard-working, responsible husband and father who has no vices. I don't know anybody as nice as Jim," she says proudly.

Shirley started worrying about Jim's health the night before he saw the doctor concerning the abnormal stools. She remembers waking in the middle of the night to find him missing from their bed. As she recalls, "He went into the bathroom and it seemed like he was in there a long time. When he climbed back in bed, his entire body felt cold." Jim doesn't know if he was cold from fear or from loss of blood. But he made an appointment immediately the next morning to see his family doctor. After running several tests, the doctor put Jim in the hospital. Two days later, they operated.

Five days passed, and Jim was still in the dark regarding the outcome of his surgery. He had asked to see the surgeon but was told they were waiting for the pathologist's report. Jim was starting to suspect there was something seriously wrong with him. As he remembers, "My family doctor finally showed up on the fifth day. He walked in my room with an intern and said, 'Well, we found out you have cancer,' and walked out of the room. He just said it and left."

Shirley was out of the room at the time. When she returned, she found Jim in tears. "After Jim told me what had happened, I was beside myself with anger." Jim had been left alone to absorb a totally unexpected cancer diagnosis. How did he feel? He admits, "I was upset, of course, but what could I do?"

Lothair

Lothair, a product of strong German-Lutheran stock, remembers feeling quite calm after learning his prostate was cancerous. "I look at myself and I marvel at how this thing didn't even faze me when the doctor told me I had cancer."After 65 years of practiced self-discipline, trim, well-groomed Lothair would have been expected to react as he did. Born and raised in St. Paul, Lothair grew up in a very religious environment and attended a Lutheran parochial school.

At the age of 11, Lothair fell in love for the first time—with the violin. He won a Schubert Club scholarship and organized a string trio in high school. His wife Ruth, who played cello in the trio, will vouch for his talent. "That's why I fell for him; he played the violin so beautifully. I have always told him that if he stops playing the violin, I'll leave him." Even in high school, Lothair's social life continued to be centered in the church. He and Ruth both became active in several church-sponsored organizations and still maintain close friendships with couples they met at that time.

After high school, Lothair briefly attended the University of Minnesota and then enlisted in the Air Force. The country was in the midst of World War II, and he found the military environment stifling. Thanks to his electronic expertise, he was put in charge of electronic maintenance at a twin-engine training base in Arizona.

He and Ruth were married in Arizona and returned to Minnesota shortly before the end of the war. Lothair's musical background opened up an opportunity for him to get in on the ground floor of the original magnetic tape products group at 3M in St. Paul. "I had the golden ear they were looking for," Lothair remembers. He would make recordings, listen to them, and select those that would be used for selling the magnetic tape to radio stations. Thirty-three years after joining 3M, he retired with a full pension.

Lothair then began devoting hours of time and energy to his new vocation as a securities representative. Five years later, he felt his energy waning. During a trip to Colorado to visit their son, Lothair noticed he was "running out of gas." He attributed his fatigue to the altitude. When he returned home, he saw his family doctor, who guessed it was the five-week flu and started Lothair on antibiotics. They didn't help, and things went even further downhill. Additional blood tests showed nothing.

Lothair and Ruth decided it was time to head for the Mayo Clinic, where he had been treated successfully for gallstones several years earlier. On first examination, Mayo doctors suspected prostate problems and scheduled a series of tests for later in the month. "Four weeks later, I started going through the tests. Whether a month could have made a difference, I don't know."

The tests confirmed problems with the prostate. Lothair remembers the doctor telling him, "You know, you're not just getting old and stiff like you say. I think you've got a more serious problem." The probable diagnosis was cancer of the prostate. Surgery confirmed the diagnosis, and by now, the cancer had spread to his bones.

Malinda

When Malinda enters a room, heads turn. Her dark auburn hair is cut short and settles in wisps across high cheekbones. An ever-present smile displays a row of perfect teeth set against deep rose lipstick. Her soft cowl-neck sweater, the same deep rose as her lips, hides any evidence of Malinda's cancer.

In a quiet Missouri twang, she explains the chemo pack she wears on her belt. For the next 48 hours, a small pump within the pack will feed chemicals up a tube and into the vein near her heart. After undergoing a modified radical mastectomy two years ago at the age of 28, Malinda's breast cancer has recently metastasized to her bones.

Until her cancer came along and surprised them, Malinda's entire family had been untouched by major illness. She says, "I'm the oldest of four children, and the oldest of all the grandchildren, too. This is the first time anyone in my family has had cancer. That was part of the surprise."

When Malinda was born, her father was farming, but he soon went into agribusiness and the family moved often. "That's what I thought was normal," she remembers, "to move every one or two years. Whenever the refrigerator needed defrosting, we moved."

After high school, she attended college and graduated from the University of Missouri with a degree in art. Malinda's primary talent is in three-dimensional work—pottery and sculpture. She recalls her college years: "I started out in drafting, but that was in the era when girls didn't go into architecture. I had started taking some architectural and drafting classes, but I was the only girl and felt out of place." So she channeled her energies into an art major.

After graduation, Malinda taught seventh and eighth grade art in St. Joseph, Missouri, a job she loved. She enjoyed working with the teenagers and also enjoyed having the summer off to work on her own art.

After she married, her husband's work took them to Minneapolis. Malinda was unable to find another teaching position. She took a course on working opportunities for women, then chose to put her artistic flare to work for her in a sales position. She became a manager in a large department store.

During the next three years, her husband changed jobs three times. They moved to Kansas City and then back to Minneapolis. "Every time he moved, I just tried to find something to do. You know, good old dutiful wife. When we moved back from Kansas City, I was the one who had to stay behind and get the moving van and all that business."

Once settled back in Minneapolis, Malinda took a sales job with the Hoover Vacuum Cleaner Company. She became their star pupil and was promoted after only six months. She was responsible for selling the products to dealers and following up to help them promote the product to the customer.

She was successful, and she was enjoying herself. Remembering those times, she says, "I was 28, in good health, and had a good job. I thought things were going well for me. I thought I had all the things you're supposed to have in life." Malinda gestures with her hands as if to place quotation marks around "supposed to have."

One month after receiving her promotion, while going through a physical workout in the morning, Malinda noticed a firmness in the upper part of her right breast. As she describes it, "It was hard as a rock. I would run and my breast wouldn't move. I just thought my exercise program was working and firming me up."

But she worried about the firmness and two weeks later she saw a doctor. The doctor thought it was highly unusual but didn't know what it was. Malinda assured him she wasn't pregnant. He asked her to come back in a month. "He said that with women and their breasts, it often is the result of hormones. But he really didn't know," she says.

Within a month's time, the whole upper half of the breast was involved. Malinda returned to the same doctor. This time he sent her for a mammogram immediately. Malinda was getting worried. "The X-ray technician said, 'Wow! Is your breast ever hard.' First of all, I didn't expect that from some technician. Secondly, I started thinking maybe she hadn't seen anything like this before. Now I was even more nervous."

Suddenly, things started happening faster than Malinda expected. She had the mammogram on a Friday. At 6:30 that evening, the doctor called. He had taken the liberty of sending the mammograms to another doctor for a second opinion.

Malinda was scheduled for an appointment with the surgeon first thing Monday morning.

She and her husband spent a tearful, nerve-racking weekend. "The fact they were being so serious made us realize we had to be serious about this too," she admits. On Monday, they both went to see the second doctor, a surgeon with a specialty in oncology. She recalls painfully: "After about a three-minute palpation, the doctor told me to put my clothes on and he would get my husband. That was all it took. He told us he was 99 percent certain it was cancer, and from feeling the lymph nodes he was convinced it had started to spread."

Two days later, Malinda's surgeon removed her right breast and 20 cancerous lymph nodes. "When he first told me it was cancer, I thought, I'm going to die. I didn't know many people with cancer. But the people I did know had all died."

Bill

Bill, a handsome young man in his early thirties, grew up in a family of achievers. When he greets you with a firm handshake and a genuinely warm smile, you feel as if you have known him all your life. He maintains constant eye contact as he tells you his story. He is obviously at ease with himself and with life.

Bill lived most of his young life on a farm near Fairmont, Minnesota. As he tells it, "My dad was an important person in Fairmont. You know, being president of the 3M plant in town meant you were involved in everything. He was on the Boy Scout board, the bank board, the hospital board. You name it, he did it." Bill's mother was also active. Besides bringing up four children, his mother was involved in the Girl Scouts and in the American Association of University Women. She was a registered nurse.

When Bill was a junior in high school, his father was transferred back to St. Paul. Bill finished high school in Mahtomedi and decided against going to college. His older brother John was working at a golf course at the time. When the management of the golf course wanted some stumps removed, Bill and John decided to go into business for themselves.

"John knew we could buy the stump removal machine for $5,000," Bill recalled. "So Dad challenged us. He said if we could prove we could make money at it, he would invest. He bought the machine, and we paid him back."

Being involved in an occupation that allowed him to be outdoors on some sort of machine was perfect for Bill. Since childhood, he had loved machines—the faster, the better. "That's me," he confessed. "Snowmobiles, three wheelers, motorcycles. I've always got to test them out and see how fast they'll go. Dad claims I'm always getting hurt." After two broken arms and a broken wrist, Bill proved his dad was right. The next winter, Bill expanded his business to include snowplowing. "You needed four-wheel drive for the stump machine. Why not hang a plow on the front and use it in the winter?"

Bill had been in business about five years when he began having physical problems. He started seeing a doctor because he had a swollen testicle. The doctor gave him an antibiotic, but it didn't seem to do anything. Bill then saw a specialist, who gave him more antibiotics. But the testicle remained swollen and sore. The doctor suggested it might be cancer and encouraged Bill to go in for surgery right away. Bill's dad had always preached to him that "knowledge is power," so he sought a second opinion before making his decision. After receiving concurring opinions from other doctors, Bill agreed to immediate surgery.

The surgeon removed the testicle and Bill went home the same day. Three days later he went in for a few more tests, including a CT scan. As he remembers, he was feeling pretty good. "After the tests, I still felt well enough to go sit on the stump machine and do some work." Bill stopped by his parents' house at three that afternoon to pick up any phone messages.

His mom and dad grabbed him the minute he walked in the door. The hospital had already called. It was cancer, and he had another tumor the size of an orange growing next to his liver and kidney. The doctors wanted him back in the hospital by six o'clock that night to do surgery in the morning.

Bill was scared. When he got in his car, the tears came. He couldn't believe he had to be back in the hospital in less than three hours. He wanted to talk to friends before checking in.

As Bill recalls, his drive to a friend's house was terrifying. "I can remember hanging onto that steering wheel with my mind racing a mile a minute. My hands were just sweating. The next thing I knew, I glanced down at the speedometer, and the needle was all the way to the right. I said to myself, 'Wait a minute. You're not dead yet. No sense killing yourself.'"

Lou

Lou speaks clearly and calmly when she introduces herself, but what you hear is a real earful. "I started with ovarian cancer many years ago," she recounts. "After my surgery, I had several good years. Then the cancer recurred in the liver. Now it has spread to my bones, and I have a few spots on my lungs."

Sounds bad? You wouldn't think so if you met Lou face to face. It's hard to remember what strikes you first about her. Is it her almost iridescent white hair, or is it her piercing blue eyes? Either way, in between is a perfect complexion and an almost constant smile. She appears healthy and vibrant, despite the fact that her cancer is actively growing and will probably never be cured.

A beautiful handmade tapestry depicting Iceland and its many customs is displayed prominently on a wall in Lou and her husband Ingvar's living room. That single piece of embroidery tells you a great deal about Lou. She says, "I worked almost nonstop for days to complete that piece. I would go from room to room following the sun so I would have the best light to work. One day

Ingvar came home, and I hadn't even changed out of my bed clothes. I was dedicated to getting it done."

Both Lou and Ingvar speak in a heavy Icelandic brogue, and their heritage is obviously an important part of their life. "Our grandparents immigrated to a small Icelandic community about sixty miles north of Winnipeg. We were both very close to our grandparents. Ingvar was even confirmed in Icelandic. Our grand-parents had been very good friends in Iceland before they left for Canada."

Lou and Ingvar grew up together. Because he is five years older than she is, they didn't really notice each other when they were young. But as they grew older, something happened. "I had always known this fellow," she says, looking at him fondly. "But all of a sudden, I don't know what blossomed out, but it did." Before Ingvar left to go in the service, he gave Lou an engagement ring. "I trusted she would wait for me, but I thought the ring would help," Ingvar adds. Lou went into nurses' training at Winnipeg General Hospital. And she waited for Ingvar to return.

After Lou graduated and Ingvar returned home, they married and started a family. A few years later, they moved to the United States. Lou says: "My sister and her husband had just moved to Newport, Minnesota. She told me about the nursing opportunities. Things weren't that promising in Canada." Lou went ahead with their small son. Once in Minnesota, she recognized opportunities for Ingvar. As luck would have it, he signed on at 3M. Ingvar remembers, "I started as a helper at 3M and was fortunate enough to become an apprentice machinist. When I applied, I was con-vinced I would never hear from them." He did hear from them and spent 31 years as a machinist.

Lou's sister was already working at St. John's Hospital. Her reputation made it easy for Lou to find work there also. "My sis-ter's supervisor told her that if I was half as good as she was, I would be hired." She was hired without an interview.

When their second boy was born, Lou decided to stay home full time for four years to take care of the boys. She then returned to the working world as a school nurse in St. Paul Park. Ingvar remembers how dedicated Lou was through those years. "When she was a school nurse, Lou and another woman had 6,000 children to look after. Lou would bring the work home—all the reports. Sometimes the parents would act like they didn't care. That would bother her. All this added up."

Lou admits that she let the pressures of the job get to her. "Those six years I was a school nurse, I fought with a duodenal ulcer. I'm that kind of person. I can get real uptight. Looking back, I know I took many things too seriously. I shouldn't have been bringing my work home and calling parents at night. Yet I felt a sense of responsibility for all those kids."

But when one of her ovaries ruptured, Lou had to start focusing on herself. "Before it happened, I had had problems with pain. My gynecologist had told me there was nothing to worry about. He thought I had an inflamed ovary, so I just put up with it. Sometimes I would have such pain, I thought everything was going to fall out." Finally, in December, she was rushed to the hospital. They operated immediately, and Lou was put in intensive care. The results came two days later.

"The doctor talked to us very frankly. He said I had a slow-growing cancer. He tried to clean it all out, but there were bits and pieces left. He said I could live for two years, or I could live for 20 years. At the time, Bruce was only 14 years old. I thought to myself, oh my God. This kid is so young. I've got to live to see him graduate from high school. A boy needs his mother at least that long."

John and Hazel

By the time John got the call telling him the growth on his colon was malignant, he was prepared. He had been introduced to cancer four years earlier when his wife Hazel had a malignant lump removed from her breast.

Today, after 55 years of marriage, John and Hazel are both free of cancer. John pours a cup of coffee and makes himself comfortable on his recently built screen porch. Their 50-year-old Stillwater home has seen four children grow up and is a second home to nine grandchildren. At 75, John has been retired 12 years. But that doesn't mean he's bored. "I retired at 63, and I've been busy every day since," he says proudly. John's woodwork is on display all over the house—Christmas ornaments, nativity scenes, message boards, even a dice game. With a workshop behind his garage and another in his basement, John spends a part of each day on wood projects. He and Hazel sell most of what he makes at craft fairs.

John's constant good humor is evident when he laughingly makes fun of himself. He is known for his post-retirement habit of sleeping until almost noon. "I start late and quit early, so I don't get much done. But this is a hobby, not a job. I like what I do, but I don't want to stay at it steady eight hours a day like when I was working."

John spent 36 years in the purchasing department of a shoe company in Stillwater. He loved his work. Then, when he was 57, the company closed its doors. "They gave me my last check and said goodbye," he recalls ruefully. For the next six years, he worked at a sheet metal company until his retirement.

When his wife, Hazel, found a lump in her breast, she saw the doctor immediately and had surgery two days later. The olive-sized lump was malignant, and Hazel lost the entire breast. "When I came to and found the breast gone, I knew immediately what it was," she recalls. "That really scared me. It was a shock finding nothing there at all." She knew very little about cancer, and she was afraid. "Our hospital was offering I CAN COPE classes for the first time soon after that," she remembered. "It was John who finally convinced me we both should go."

After the classes ended, John and Hazel continued attending a cancer support group once a week. Four years later, in mid-January, John noticed blood in his stool. "I went directly to the phone and called the doctor." The next day, the doctor did a proctoscope and found a half-inch growth. He sent a tissue sample to the lab and told John he would get back to him in a few days.

Three days later, the results were in. The growth was malignant. But John wasn't afraid. "Through Hazel's support group, I had met many people already who had had colon cancer and were getting along fine. That's the direction I wanted to go. I was going to be like them."

The Aftermath

The day the doctor confirmed their cancer was not an easy one for any of these people. The surprise and the shock of the diagnosis numbed them. For many, that shock was magnified by postoperative weakness and vulnerability. The first common thread woven through the reactions of almost all people with cancer, regardless of age, is usually disbelief. They had known something was wrong. But not cancer. Not me. "It was devastating to find out I had cancer," said Malinda. "That's the first thing I remember—just being so shocked."

Hearing the diagnosis is a shock. Most people experience feelings of numbness, raw fear, or paralysis. For some, those emotions last for hours; for others, days and weeks. Suddenly they are facing a variety of losses. Loss of income. Loss of health. Loss of love and support. Perhaps loss of life. That first encounter with the disease is a time of turmoil.

Coming to grips with that turmoil is seldom a neat and orderly process. It is more like a hurricane. People are tossed about by waves of emotion—anger, denial, depression. Periods of calm set in only to be followed by another surge of panic. Usually the greatest panic is borne of fear.

After hearing the words "You have cancer," people are afraid of many things: fear of cancer itself, often considered the most dreaded affliction in America; fear of the unknown; fear of death. Except for Dave, whose younger sister had died of cancer many years earlier, few knew what to expect. Most of these people knew little or nothing about cancer. Malinda believed that anyone who has cancer dies. Lothair worried about the pain. Dick feared permanent disability.

Family and friends are afraid, too. Their reactions often intensify the anxiety of the people with cancer and make their own fears stronger. Jim's wife, Shirley, vividly recalled her father's five-year bout with cancer and his eventual death. Those memories fueled her own fears. Now, being confronted with Jim's mortality, she was also aware of her own eventual death.

As fear and panic wane and reality is internalized, people are ready to start reassessing their lives in preparation for rebuilding. That rebuilding means finding a balance somewhere between denial and totally giving up. Author Cornelius Ryan says it well when he speaks of his own reaction to prostate cancer. In his book *A Private Battle,* he writes, "My mind swings from disbelief to fatalism. I am vacillating between a surging belief that all will be well and a maudlin conviction that nothing will ever be right again."

Some days, Ryan found himself giving in to death. Other days, he totally denied the seriousness of his condition. Both feelings are natural and can be expected as people with cancer attempt to come to grips with their diagnosis. To stay healthy with cancer, people need to find a balance somewhere between these two extremes. Finding that balance is easier when people are able to learn more about cancer and when they have the loving support of others who care.

The journey toward acceptance begins the minute the diagnosis is presented. How it is presented has an impact on how people perceive their cancer. In Bill's case, being summoned to the hospital for more surgery the next day was extremely frightening. The message he got was that there was no time to waste. That meant his condition was serious. His longtime family physician found it difficult to break the bad news of cancer to Jim. As a result, Jim received his diagnosis alone, and in a less-than-empathetic manner. Debbie's surgeon actually downplayed the seriousness of her condition by calling it a "form of cancer." The result was that Debbie felt lucky, partly because she didn't know any better.

Information is power. What you don't know has power over you. Lack of knowledge regarding cancer and its treatment can render the person with cancer powerless. If you don't know anything about your disease, how do you know what to do about it? Who do you ask? Who do you trust?

Harry Truman had three stamps on his desk: "Yes," "No," and "Need More Information." If he had any doubt about how to proceed, he delayed his decision and used the third stamp. People with cancer need to concentrate on using this third stamp before making crucial decisions about their health and their life. Those decisions can't be made without good information.

Questions pop up all the time. What exactly is cancer? How long have I had it? Why did I get it? How will you treat me? For how long? Will I be sick? Will I die? No one has all the answers. Cancer is more than one disease, and every type of cancer has its own set of problems and questions. I CAN COPE was designed to cover the most common concerns and answer the questions most often asked.

But the person with cancer must answer the most difficult question. Will I learn to live with cancer? Or will I give up? The people you have met have started the long process of learning how to help themselves. They are beginning to live for today.

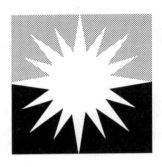

"There is no type of cancer

for which there is

no treatment;

and there is

no type of cancer

from which some people

have not been cured."

Richard Bloch
Fighting Cancer

CHAPTER ONE

Learning About Cancer

In Chinese, the word crisis is written with two characters. The first symbol represents danger. The second means opportunity. The relationship between danger and opportunity is roughly equivalent to the relationship between cancer and health. People who refer to themselves as "cancer victims" are stuck in the danger mode of crisis, unable to see their choices—their opportunities. Immobilized by fear, they have difficulty pulling themselves together.

On the other hand, getting past the danger mode to the opportunity mode opens new channels. Cancer veterans talk about regrowth, about getting priorities straight, about coming through the experience a better person with a clearer vision of life. When people are given the tools to identify options and make informed choices, they can move from being passive cancer victims into the role of active cancer patients.

When Jim's doctor broke the news, he announced that Jim had cancer—nothing more. The doctor said the dreaded word but failed to follow up with the necessary information. This left Jim and his family in the danger mode. Thankfully, Jim remembers, the nursing staff came to the rescue: "When the head nurse came in the room, our whole family was in tears. We were devastated. We didn't know anything about cancer. Then the nurse started telling us what treatments were available. The more we knew, the better we felt."

Knowledge is power. That power can open the door to hope. To make choices and assume control, Jim and his family needed to know more about the disease that had taken them by surprise. The first step is understanding the basic nature of cancer.

Introducing Cancer

Cancer—One Word, Many Diseases

Cancer. This one word represents not one, but more than 150 different types of disease. Cancer can occur in almost every part of the body. Each cancer has unique characteristics and its own unique treatment. According to one theory, all cancer starts from a single cell. Whether it is in the breast, lung, colon, or blood, at some point a single, normal cell goes through a dramatic transformation and becomes a cancer cell.

Abnormal Versus Normal Cell Growth

The body is made up of billions of cells, and each cell reproduces itself by dividing. This constant cell division allows for the growth and repair of body tissues and is a normal, healthy process. When that growth or repair is complete, a set of genes tells the body to "switch off" the process, and cell growth stops. But cancer cells have a mind of their own. They have no thermostatic gene to switch them off. A change in their genetic code makes cancer cells "forget" to stop growing. The once-normal cell becomes abnormal, and it behaves erratically rather than predictively. Cell division becomes uncontrolled; the cells go on a rampage and multiply at a wild rate rather than dividing normally. This abnormal cell growth eventually forms a cell cluster called a tumor.

Benign Versus Malignant Tumors

A tumor can be classified as either benign or malignant. A benign tumor is not cancerous. Fortunately, most tumors are benign. Although it may grow large, a benign tumor will not spread to other parts of the body. Usually it can be removed with little chance for recurrence.

A malignant tumor is cancerous and can invade surrounding tissue. The uncontrolled growth of the cancerous tumor eventually crowds out healthy cells. In addition, cells of the cancerous tumor can split off and travel through the body via the blood or lymph systems to form tumors in new locations. This process is called metastasis. For this reason, cancer can recur even after the tumor itself has been surgically removed.

Types of Cancer

A solid tumor is classified as either a carcinoma or a sarcoma. Carcinomas are the most common type of tumor, representing about 85 percent of all cancers. These develop in the epithelium, the tissue lining internal organs and passageways. Cancers of the skin, lung, breast, colon, and uterus are examples of carcinomas. Sarcomas are soft tissue tumors arising in the connective tissue, muscles, or bones. Jim's tumor was diagnosed as leiomyosarcoma, a rare cancer of the connective tissue. In Jim's case, it was the connective tissue surrounding his stomach. Although this type of cancer can metastasize through the blood, there was no initial indication in Jim's case that a metastasis had occurred.

Blood-forming tumors are the second major form of cancer. These tumors include myeloma, leukemia, and lymphoma. Myelomas arise in blood plasma cells, which are part of the bone marrow. Multiple myeloma invades the marrow and destroys normal bone. Leukemia is also a cancer of blood-forming tissues, but it is characterized by an overproduction of white blood cells. Lymphomas arise in the cells of the lymph system. The lymph glands (or nodes) are small, round, or bean-shaped structures found throughout the body and are a major site of response against infection. Lymph is a clear fluid that drains from all body tissue through the nodes, which are found in the neck, groin, armpits, and spleen. Bacteria and other foreign objects are trapped and destroyed in these glands, which usually swell when reacting to something foreign. Tumor cells that break away from a primary tumor often localize in the lymph nodes. Hodgkin's disease is a form of lymphoma.

Who Gets Cancer–And Why

Cancer can be called an equal-opportunity disease. It develops in people of all ages, races, and ethnic backgrounds. About one in three people today will eventually get some form of cancer. In the United States, approximately 1.2 million new cases are diagnosed each year. Over 8 million Americans alive today have a history of cancer, with about 4 million of these diagnosed five or more years ago. Most of these 4 million can be considered cured.

Men and women over 55 years of age make up the largest cancer population. While cancer is rare in children and young adults, it does occur. Leukemia is the most common form of childhood cancer, followed by cancers of the central nervous system. Young people up to the age of 20 are among the group most likely to get cancer of the brain.

Theories about why people get cancer abound, and more are being added every year. Although the exact mechanism is still unknown, we do know what doesn't cause cancer.

Cancer is Not Contagious

In spite of the many theories about what causes cancer, researchers agree that cancer is not contagious. The disease cannot be spread by physical contact or by drinking from the same cup. Still, many people with cancer experience immense isolation and loneliness because of these unfortunate myths.

No one should be afraid to embrace or kiss a person with cancer for fear of "catching" it. To the contrary, love and affection are needed now more than ever. A person's cancer is as unique as that person's genes. To think you can catch someone else's cancer is as far fetched as thinking you can catch that person's hair color.

Injuries Don't Cause Cancer

Some people believe injuries cause cancer because an injury calls attention to an existing cancer. Except for a very rare cancer, there is no evidence that cancer could be caused by an injury.

Growth of the Cancerous Cell

The formation of a cancer is a multi-step process. Within a human cell lie anywhere from 50,000 to 100,000 genes. Research suggests that perhaps no more than 100 regulate cell growth and division. As cell formation takes place, several things must happen for a cancer cell to form instead of a normal cell. If this were not so, cancer cells might be created every time someone was exposed to a potentially cancer-causing agent.

Today many scientists believe that the culprit responsible for the transformation from normal to abnormal cell growth is the oncogene ("onco" meaning tumor). But what activates the oncogene? One popular theory suggests that cancers arise from at least two different assaults, or "hits," to the genes on the cell. These assaults occur when the human body is exposed to any of the risk factors currently linked to cancer's formation.

Generally, several years elapse from the moment a microscopic cell turns cancerous until it forms a tumor large enough to cause suspicious symptoms. In fact, some cancer cells take about 100 days just to divide into two cells. At that rate, it would take the cell 8 or 9 years to develop into a solid tumor that could be felt or would show on a scan or X-ray. This is the common progression for many types of breast and colon cancer.

Some cancer cells can grow and divide much faster and take only a month or two to become a visible cancer. Although most breast cancers grow slowly, Malinda's inflammatory breast cancer was an exception. Oat cell cancer, a form of lung cancer, and some types of leukemia and lymphoma are other examples of fast-growing cancers.

Cancer Causes and Prevention

The multi-step process that leads to a cancer probably involves several cancer-causing agents working together as co-carcinogens. Pinpointing exactly what triggers a cancer is often difficult because of the multiple-hit theory and because it sometimes takes 20 years or more for a cancer to develop after exposure to a carcinogen.

John Higgenson, M.D., former director of the International Agency for Research on Cancer, once said that 70 to 90 percent of all human cancers are caused by the environment. Today, many environmental factors are suspect in cancer's formation.

Smoking

Cigarette smoking is the most harmful environmental hazard in the United States today and is the single most important element in cancer formation. Dick's 30-year smoking habit, which led to his eventual lung cancer, is just one of countless examples reminding us that smoking is definitely hazardous to your health.

Today we are in the midst of a lung cancer epidemic. A rare disease in the early 1900s, lung cancer now claims approximately 150,000 lives per year in the United States. And, whereas lung cancer used to be primarily a man's disease, women now develop it in equal numbers. Before 1987, breast cancer caused the most cancer deaths among women. But estimates for 1993 predicted 46,000 women would die of breast cancer and 56,000 would die of lung cancer. Why the change? Women today have "come a long way" and are smoking in record numbers.

The incidence of all new cancers is rising only slightly every year. However, almost all of that increase is related to tobacco smoking. If lung and voice-box cancers were removed from the statistics, cancer mortality in the United States would actually show a downward trend. And if everyone suddenly quit using tobacco, an estimated 90 percent of all lung cancers would be eliminated.

New information from the Surgeon General and the National Academy of Sciences now claims people don't have to smoke to be at risk from smoking. Studies have shown that exposure to other people's smoke increases the risk of developing lung cancer. An American Cancer Society study concluded that non-smokers exposed to 20 or more cigarettes a day had twice the risk of developing lung cancer. And adults aren't the only ones at risk.

The Environmental Protection Agency (EPA) reported that exposure to secondhand tobacco smoke accounts for tens of thousands of serious respiratory ailments each year in young children. Those under the age of 18 months face substantial risk of serious bronchitis and pneumonia, and exposure to secondary smoke also exacerbates asthmatic symptoms.

Although respiratory problems and lung cancer remain the most common ailments associated with smoking, tobacco use is also related to cancers of the lip, tongue, sinuses, pharynx, and possibly even breast and pancreas. Users of powdered tobacco (snuff) also have a greater chance of developing oral cancer. An upswing in oral cancer among young people prompted the U.S. government to outlaw television advertising for smokeless tobacco.

Clearly, a top priority of the American Cancer Society and the National Cancer Institute is to eliminate the use of tobacco. The good news is that it is never too late to stop smoking. Once a person stops, the body starts healing itself immediately, and the risk of lung cancer begins to drop. It takes years for detectable malignant changes to develop in the lung. Such changes can be arrested by prolonged abstinence from smoking—but only before the malignancy begins.

Sun

In a country of sun worshippers, where tanning parlors are popping up in every shopping center, the American public appears to be unfazed by the connection between sun and skin cancers. Yet we know that almost all of the 700,000 cases of nonmelanoma skin cancer occurring each year in the United States are sun related. Most of these are basal cell or squamous cell cancers, which are highly curable.

In addition, epidemiological studies have shown that sun exposure is a major factor in the development of melanoma, a dangerous and often uncontrollable form of cancer that starts from a flat or slightly elevated brown spot on the skin. Approximately 35,000 people are diagnosed with melanoma each year; since 1973, the incidence of melanoma in American has increased about 4 percent per year.

Overexposure to the sun's ultraviolet rays is becoming more risky with the thinning of the protective ozone layer. Fair-skinned people who freckle are more susceptible than people of color or people who tan easily. If you must be in the sun for long periods of time, use a sunscreen. Hats and other coverings should be worn whenever possible to offer maximum protection to all skin surfaces.

A simple ABCD rule spells out the warning signs of a melanoma. A is for asymmetry. One half of the mole does not match the other half. B is for border irregularity, or ragged edges. C is for color, with pigmentation that is not uniform. D is for diameter greater than 6 millimeters. Any sudden or progressive increase in size should be of special concern.

Diet

Research continues on how excesses or deficiencies in a person's diet might play a role in the cause and prevention of cancer. High-fat and low-fiber diets are of special concern. Colon, breast, and uterine cancers appear to be associated with obesity.

In addition, a high-fat diet is suspected of being a factor in development of certain cancers, particularly those of the breast, colon, and prostate.

Colon cancer, the second most common cancer in the Western world, may be partly related to the amount of fiber in the diet. Colon cancer is virtually unheard of among tribal Africans. An English researcher did extensive studies on the Bantu tribe in South Africa. The Bantu's diet consisted of a large amount of roughage, and they passed stools more frequently than is typical in Western culture. When a person is constipated, food stays in the colon longer and has a chance to interact with the tissue. This interaction may contribute to the development of cancer. The researcher concluded that roughage protects against colon cancer by forcing the stools to move through the system faster. This has not been proven, but the study suggests a definite correlation.

In addition, when people of this same tribe moved out of their native habitat and adopted Western habits, their incidence of colon cancer increased. People of color born in the United States have the same incidence of colon cancer as their white counterparts. In some cases, the rate is even higher.

This isn't absolute proof that eating a diet high in fiber will prevent colon cancer. But for certain, it is healthy in that it helps to prevent other problems such as hemorrhoids, polyps, diverticulitis, or appendicitis.

Breast cancer is the most common cancer among American women, yet it is rare in Japan. If someone of Japanese heritage is born in Hawaii, however, she has a much greater chance of breast cancer. And, if born and raised in a Western lifestyle, Japanese women are just as likely as Caucasian women to have breast cancer. Some studies have suggested that the high-fat diet most women consume in the United States is a factor in the high incidence of breast cancer.

Stomach cancer, on the other hand, has been on the decline in the United States. Yet it is a very common cancer in Japan. The

Japanese consume large quantities of smoked or salted fish. Such foods, as well as foods processed with nitrites, have been linked to esophageal and stomach cancer.

No discussion of nutrition would be complete without mentioning the role of vitamins and minerals. The most exciting data seems to be coming from studies done on beta carotene, a relative of vitamin A found in green and orange vegetables such as sweet potatoes, carrots, and dandelion greens. Early research results suggest that a diet rich in beta carotene can lower the risk of some cancers, including lung, breast, cervix, and stomach. One of the first studies reporting success in humans was conducted at the University of Arizona Cancer Center in 1989. Patients with precancerous lesions in their mouths were given 30 mg. of beta carotene daily. After three to six months, lesions in 70 percent of the patients were dramatically reduced.

Enough evidence now exists to suggest that diet plays a significant role in cancer prevention. That diet should emphasize foods that are low in fat and cholesterol and should include a daily variety of fresh fruits and vegetables. The American Cancer Society guidelines propose eating more high-fiber foods such as whole-grain cereals, breads, and pasta, since a high-fiber diet may reduce the risk of colon cancer. They also suggest cutting down on total fat intake, limiting consumption of alcohol, and avoiding salt-cured, smoked, and nitrite-cured foods. Because individuals 40 percent or more overweight increase their risk of colon, breast, prostate, gallbladder, ovary, and uterine cancers, the ACS also recommends maintaining a desirable weight.

Occupational Exposure

Environmental experts have suggested that harmful chemicals—fumes, dusts, etc.—in the workplace are probably responsible for approximately 5 percent of all cancers. Various occupational hazards, especially ionizing radiation and chemicals like asbestos, benzene, and vinyl chloride are known to cause cancer when exposure levels are high.

Industrial workers are particularly susceptible to lung diseases when exposed to the combined effect of smoking and exposure to toxic chemicals. For instance, a man who smokes and works in an asbestos plant is 60 times more likely to develop lung cancer than a man who does neither.

Other chemical agents that are suspect include arsenic, uranium, nickel, chromium, tars, and beta-naphthylamine. Fumes from rubber or chlorine could also be dangerous, as well as dust from cotton and coal.

Radiation

Survivors of the atomic bomb in Japan, the subject of several studies, show an increased incidence of leukemia and bone sarcoma. Surgeons' hands often develop skin cancer after years of exposure to radiation under a fluoroscope, and radiologists, the doctors who specialize in the use of X-rays, also show an increased incidence of leukemia. All these individuals have been exposed to high levels of radiation, which does not typify the radiation exposure of the average person. Today medical X-rays are adjusted to deliver the lowest possible dose. Despite the safety of today's diagnostic X-rays, the wise patient should ask for a certified X-ray technician, since the majority of any individual's radiation exposure will come from medical or dental procedures.

The 1979 accident at the Three Mile Island nuclear-power plant near Harrisburg, Pennsylvania, and the catastrophic 1986 explosion at the Chernobyl plant in Russia reignited public concern over the release of radiation into the environment. Near Chernobyl, the incidence of thyroid cancer, leukemia, and other radiation-related illnesses increased after the accident. While some forms of cancer show up immediately after exposure to high levels of radiation, the effects of exposure to low-level radiation are not yet known. A major concern is the potential for genetic damage. Unfortunately, the total damage done by Chernobyl will take years to assess.

More recently, radon, an odorless, colorless, radioactive gas that occurs naturally as a result of uranium formations in the environment, has been implicated in causing lung cancer among nonsmokers. Normally, this gas escapes through fissures in the earth and dissipates into the atmosphere. In the home, however, radon can seep through cracks in the foundation, sump pumps, or drains and build up within the house.

Radon levels in the home vary according to the amount coming in, the rate at which it enters, and the rate at which ventilation exhausts it out. Persons living in areas of high uranium concentration should consider having their homes tested for radon by a public agency or a private laboratory.

Radar guns, used by law-enforcement agencies, are another source of radiation that has spurred controversy in recent years. Some states banned the use of handheld speed detectors after several police officers claimed long-term exposure to the guns gave them cancer. Could a testicular cancer be the result of a radar gun being held between an officer's legs? No studies confirm or deny such a claim; the dilemma only points out the potential dangers of long-term exposure to radiation across the electromagnetic spectrum.

Electromagnetic fields (EMF) fall into the same category. Epidemiologists have been busy for several years trying to gain a better picture of whether living near high-voltage power lines increases the risk of cancer. Preliminary findings suggest a link between exposure to electromagnetic fields and cancer, specifically leukemia and cancers of the brain and breast. But the truth will not be known until researchers scientifically confirm or deny a deleterious relationship between electromagnetic fields and biological systems. Most scientists suggest "prudent avoidance" of electromagnetic fields until their effects on the human body are fully understood.

Genetic Risk Factors

Some types of cancer clearly have a familial tendency, particularly cancers of the ovaries, colon, and breast. To say that a cancer runs in the family, however, does not necessarily mean that cancer is hereditary; family tendency is only one factor among many in the disease process. An average woman in the United States has a one-in-nine chance of getting breast cancer. But if that woman's mother had breast cancer before menopause and she has a sister who had breast cancer before menopause, her chances of getting breast cancer are greatly increased. The same holds true for colon cancer. If several family members have had colon cancer, chances of another member developing that cancer are considerably higher than average. Doctors should watch high-risk individuals closely, examining them at younger ages and more often.

Having a relative with cancer shouldn't be cause for panic. And those who don't have cancer in their family tree shouldn't be overly confident. Remember, cancer formation is a multi-step process. Even though family history is a factor, it is directly responsible for only a small percentage of cancers. If you are concerned, take the following steps:

- Limit exposure to known risks.
- Heed early warning signs of cancer.
- Make sure your doctor has a thorough family history.
- Have regular checkups.
- Consider genetic counseling to estimate risk based on family medical history.

Stress, Attitude, and the Immune System– Is There a Link?

With the discovery of AIDS, a great deal of attention has been focused on the immune system's role in disease prevention. The immune system is actually a complex network of organs and tissues, with cells moving through the body via various fluids. Many factors influence the proper functioning of the immune system, which is made up of the spleen, lymph nodes, thymus gland, tonsils, adenoids, and the marrow in long bones. For instance, the system is weakened by viral infections, blood transfusions, certain drug treatments, and malnutrition. Recent studies have also shown that excessive alcohol consumption and cigarette smoking can depress the immune system.

In addition, a person's ability to handle stress has been linked to the immune system. Could this mean that a positive mental attitude strengthens the immune system? Eve Potts and Marion Morra, authors of the popular book *Choices*, suggest it does. They cite studies that show how attitude can affect the endocrine system and in turn affect some of the organs making up the immune system.

Currently, there is insufficient evidence to definitively link a positive mental attitude with a lower risk of cancer. But emotions do affect many diseases, and studies continue on the mysterious relationship between the body and the mind and how the two interact in the development of cancer.

The Importance of Early Detection

Obviously, practicing good health habits and avoiding risk factors are excellent ways of preventing cancer. But once a cancer exists, the next best thing is to have it diagnosed as early as possible. For most cancers, the cure rate is significantly higher if it is found early.

Early diagnosis requires a person to be knowledgeable about the potential signs and symptoms. Sometimes these signs are obvious and easily recognizable. Others can be detected only by medical examination or tests. The American Cancer Society has established warning signals that everyone interested in early detection needs to commit to memory:

Cancer's Seven Warning Signals

- **C**hange in bowel or bladder habits
- **A** sore that does not heal
- **U**nusual bleeding or discharge
- **T**hickening or lump in breast or elsewhere
- **I**ndigestion or difficulty in swallowing
- **O**bvious change in a wart or mole
- **N**agging cough or hoarseness

Medical Tests to Detect Cancer

About 50 years ago, Dr. Papanicolaou, a Greek physician, introduced the Pap smear. Today, it is still the most effective test doctors have for early detection of cervical cancer. A few cells are scraped from the cervix and examined under a microscope. The test is simple, painless, and extremely effective in detecting cervical cancer in its earliest stages.

Most breast cancers are found by women doing self-examination. Adult women should adopt the healthy habit of monthly breast self-examination (BSE), since estimates say 90 percent of cancerous tumors will be found through BSE. The mammogram, which uses X-rays for detecting early breast cancer, is also an effective screening test and can find a cancer before a lump can be felt. The most effective screening for breast cancer is a yearly breast examination by a doctor, a mammogram every year or two after age 40, and monthly self-examination.

Testicular self-examination (TSE) is also a simple, effective procedure for early detection of cancer of the testes, a common cancer in men 15 to 34 years of age. As in Bill's case, this type of cancer can be treated promptly and effectively if it is discovered in the early stages. Men who have undescended or partially descended testicles are at a much higher risk of developing testicular cancer than others.

The American Cancer Society and various professional groups don't unanimously agree on screening guidelines. Keep in mind that each individual case is different, and screening should be based on the risk factors already identified. Some tests are very expensive, and the chance for error always exists.

For example, researchers at the Mayo Clinic found that the popular Hemocult (blood stool) test failed to detect more than 70 percent of colorectal cancers. Yet this test has been used as a screening tool for more than 20 years, and information from the University of Minnesota shows decreased mortality in persons consistently using the test. The American Cancer Society still considers it to be the best available means of inexpensively screening large numbers of people for colon cancer.

Controversy also surrounds another blood test used to screen for prostate cancer, the prostate-specific antigen (PSA). Proponents of the test as a screening device claim the PSA significantly increases the chance for cure by finding early cancers that are undetectable on the digital rectal exam. Opponents say the test is not specific enough, it identifies benign prostate conditions as well as malignant tumors, and the tumors it identifies in many cases would never cause real problems for the patient.

Researchers agree that some prostate cancers are virtually harmless and hope a current 16-year, $87-million study will provide valuable information on early detection and perhaps identify genetic differences between the inert form and the more hostile prostate cancers. Clinical trials are currently evaluating radical prostatectomy versus radiotherapy, chemotherapy versus observation after radiotherapy, and hormone manipulation versus observation after radical prostatectomy.

Despite the controversy over cost versus benefit, those who find an early cancer based on one of these screening tests might argue that the cost is insignificant compared with the extra years of life they may be afforded.

Screening Recommendations

Breast cancer: After age 40, an annual exam by a doctor, monthly self-exam, and a mammogram every one to two years for women 40 to 49 and yearly for those 50 and over.

Colon cancer: After age 40, a yearly digital rectal exam and test for hidden blood in the stool. After age 50, a flexible sigmoidoscopy every three to five years.

Lung cancer: An elective yearly chest X-ray after age 40, especially for smokers.

Ovarian cancer: Yearly pelvic examination for all women; pelvic ultrasound and the serum CA-125 test for women at high risk because of a strong family history of ovarian cancer.

Prostate cancer: Yearly digital rectal examination, serum chemistry profile, and a prostate specific antigen (PSA) test.

Unfortunately, there are not enough good screening tests for most cancers. And although many consider it useful, the practice of screening healthy people has not been widely accepted by the medical community or by insurance companies and third-party payors. Much more research is needed to discover screening tests that are safe, cost effective, and reliable.

Cancer Is a Chronic Illness–Not a Death Sentence

To most people, the word cancer is synonymous with death. A study done several years ago asked Americans what they feared most. Cancer was far and away the number one fear. Death was number two! Actually fear of cancer is greatly out of proportion to the true danger of the disease, especially when you consider the scientific advances resulting in better cure rates every year.

The American Cancer Society classifies cancer as a chronic illness in the same category as diabetes or heart disease. A chronic illness is defined as a permanent condition that may leave someone with a residual disability requiring rehabilitation and ongoing supervision. About 452,000 Americans who get cancer this year will be alive five years after diagnosis, a survival rate of 51 percent. But even people who are "cured" still need lifelong surveillance. The most important consideration for many cancer patients is not dying, but learning a new way of living.

People with chronic illness quickly learn the meaning of the word "wait." They wait for doctor's appointments. Wait for tests. Wait for therapy. Wait for results. And most important, they wait for some sign that their cancer has recurred. Faced with a finite amount of time, they learn to become less structured and more spontaneous. Values and priorities change. Things that used to seem important recede into the background. Short-term goals replace long-term dreams. The uncertainty surrounding chronic illness makes celebrating the temporary just that much more important.

Lou is a good example of someone coping with cancer as a chronic illness. Since the age of 30, she has had periodic recurrences of her ovarian cancer. Some years, the cancer and its treatment slowed her down considerably. Other years have been rich and productive.

Not everyone diagnosed with cancer dies of cancer. Today, with early detection, many will be cured. And advances in treatment delivery and pain control mean a better quality of life for those whose cancer can be controlled. Some people will die because we don't know enough about their cancer to cure them. Others will die simply because they didn't consult a doctor soon enough.

Cancer can lie dormant for months or years before reappearing. For many people, those months and years become a quest to find a positive outcome from what started out as a negative event. Life doesn't have to end with a diagnosis of cancer. Instead, it can take on brilliance and urgency as people strive to make meaning out of chaos.

Learning About Cancer: The Personal Stories

Hodgkin's Disease

Hodgkin's and non-Hodgkin's lymphoma combined account for only 6 percent of newly diagnosed cancers each year, with Hodgkin's disease accounting for only 20 percent of all lymphomas. In 1993, approximately 7,900 cases of Hodgkin's disease and 43,000 cases of non-Hodgkin's lymphoma were diagnosed in the United States. In its early stages, Hodgkin's disease is now a very curable cancer. The 30-year trend from the 1950s to the 1980s found deaths from Hodgkin's disease down 67 percent, and the five-year survival rate for Stage I Hodgkin's is now about 90 percent.

Dave's Hodgkin's disease had progressed well past Stage I by the time he was diagnosed. Today he wishes he would have better understood his body's early warning signs. But he didn't have persistent, painless swelling of lymph nodes in the neck or underarms, a symptom that often sends people to their doctors. And his rheumatoid arthritis diagnosis explained away the body aches and pains Dave was experiencing. Now he even wonders if all the pain medications he was taking for the arthritis might not have masked other Hodgkin's symptoms.

Dave remembers feeling more relieved than shocked when he was finally diagnosed. After all, his symptoms had been escalating for more than a year, and the final series of invasive gastrointestinal testing had been almost more than he could handle. "After I learned what it was, the symptoms actually abated a little," Dave comments. The stress of not knowing what was wrong in his body had actually made his symptoms seem more pronounced.

Once the diagnosis was made, Dave could retrace the events of the past two years and view them with the clear vision of hindsight. Cancer should have always been a consideration, since his sister Diane died of melanoma when she was 27, and two of his cousins also have cancer. And he had classic Hodgkin's disease symptoms, starting with night sweats and alcohol intolerance for more than a year before the official diagnosis.

But throughout that time, Dave's optimism had prevailed, optimism that later became his strongest coping tool. "I always believed that all these symptoms would eventually just go away on their own," he says. Unfortunately, they didn't go away. And Dave's delayed diagnosis haunts him and his wife. They have many unanswered questions. Did Dave really have rheumatoid arthritis, the disease his doctor treated for more than a year before the cancer diagnosis? Why did it take a year and a half and several doctors to identify the cancer? How long would the agony have gone on if they hadn't asked a trusted surgeon friend to take a look?

Reviewing these questions over and over won't change Dave's situation. But he hopes his story will convince others to watch for disease symptoms, listen to the body's internal warning system, and take the lead by doing independent research and by finding a caring physician to analyze the symptoms, link them with your history and habits, and do appropriate diagnostic tests.

The night sweats that plagued Dave for more than a year could have been a tipoff, had he known what they meant. But Dave, the eternal optimist, dismissed them as unimportant. "People need to realize that these kinds of symptoms aren't normal, no matter how much they want to deny it's something serious," Dave finally had to admit. The underarm lymph node the surgeon biopsied was unremarkable; Dave hadn't even noticed it.

"When I was finally diagnosed, my window of opportunity regarding treatment choices was pretty much shut," Dave muses. By then, his disease had advanced to Stage IV, with widespread organ involvement, including his bone marrow. Dave's only choice was to begin a year-long course of chemotherapy. Six months after completing his final drug treatment, the Hodgkin's disease returned. His oncologist put it bluntly: Dave could have more chemotherapy, but the chance of another recurrence was great. His only real chance for cure or long-term remission was a bone marrow transplant. "That sounded scary," Dave admits. "I didn't know anything about bone marrow transplant, and the thought of going through one was frightening."

Lung Cancer

Ironically, the number one cancer killer among men and women alike is often preventable. As early as 1950, researchers recognized that cigarette smoking was linked to cancer of the lung. But that wasn't publicized in the lay press until 1964. Fourteen years elapsed before a known cancer hazard was made public.

Approximately 170,000 new cases of lung cancer are reported in the U.S. each year, making this disease the number one cause of cancer deaths in both men and women. Cigarette smoking is the culprit in 87 percent of those deaths. However, the 1989 Surgeon General's report gave promising news: the prevalence of smoking has decreased from 40 percent in 1965 to 29 percent in 1987. Between 1964 and 1985, approximately three-quarters of a million smoking-related deaths were avoided or postponed because people either decided to quit smoking or decided not to start.

Dick was one of the lucky ones. When the surgeon found Dick's cancer, it was still in the first stage and had not metastasized to the lymph nodes. Generally, 70 to 80 percent of lung cancer patients have metastases by the time their cancer is diagnosed. Dick says, "I was just lucky. My fellow workers and my family were raising such an uproar about my cough, I didn't have any choice but to see a doctor."

Again, Dick proved that early diagnosis is a major factor in cancer survival rates. Only 13 percent of people with his type of lung cancer live five or more years after diagnosis. The rate improves dramatically to 40 percent when the cancer is detected at an early stage. Dick admits, "With my grandma and my dad both dying of cancer, and me smoking for 30 years, I shouldn't have been surprised when I learned what I had."

Dick quit smoking one year before he noticed any symptoms. He likes to believe that slowed the growth of his tumor. In addition, a baseline chest X-ray that same year made it possible to see subtle changes on his follow-up X-ray a year later. Prompt attention to symptoms, smoking cessation, and regular checkups with proper screenings made Dick one of the winners in the lung cancer battle.

His follow-up care, chemotherapy plus radiation to his brain, seemed extreme to him at the time. Ten years later, he understands more clearly the benefit of that kind of extreme treatment. He says that missing most of one lung hasn't slowed him down, and he certainly doesn't miss smoking. "Oh, I dream about it once in a while," he admits. "Then I wake up in a cold sweat, feeling like an alcoholic who just fell off the wagon. I'm thankful I quit when I did. They say it's never too late. But for me, it almost was."

Breast Cancer

Approximately one woman in nine will develop breast cancer sometime in her life. Malinda was one of them, although she didn't fit the typical breast cancer profile. Most women who develop this cancer are over 50, have a personal or family history of breast cancer, have never had children, or had their first child after age 30.

Malinda wasn't even 30 yet. "I'm the first one in our entire family to even be sick, much less the first one to show up with cancer," she recalls. "No one would believe it at first. You just don't think of someone less than 30 years old developing breast cancer."

Malinda discovered her cancer through self-examination, which is the way 90 percent of women discover a lump. For Malinda, it wasn't really a lump. As she tells it: "The first doctor I saw didn't know what to make of it. But instead of pursuing it, he simply asked me to come back in a month. During that time, I went to the library and read about it. Although my breast felt hard, I couldn't really feel a lump. It didn't sound like breast cancer to me, so I didn't worry about it."

A month later, when her doctor finally sent her for a mammogram, the whole upper breast was reddened and hard. The mammogram, a low-dose X-ray examination, is used both as a diagnostic tool and as a method of verification when a tumor is suspected. Once a breast lump is found, mammography can be effective in determining if there are other lesions too small to be felt in the same or opposite breast. But mammograms can also be misleading. What may look benign can turn out to be malignant. Tumors sometimes aren't visible when imaging young, dense breast tissue.

Because of Malinda's age, the denseness of her breast tissue, and the type of cancer, her mammogram was unclear. Her case is a good example of how the mammogram is most effective in combination with a thorough breast exam. The surgeon who examined Malinda after the mammogram, and who later performed her surgery, specialized in oncology. Just by observing and palpating the hardened, pinkish surface of her breast, he immediately recognized the symptoms of inflammatory breast cancer, a rare and fast-growing disease. The warmth of her skin suggested that tumor cells had already spread into many of her lymphatic vessels.

Malinda wondered out loud why her first doctor hadn't been more suspicious of the abnormality. "I kept thinking to myself, why didn't he know?" He didn't know because he had never seen the disease before. He guessed she had some type of infection. He chose to just "watch it," famous last words for many women. Through this experience, Malinda learned a difficult, but important, lesson. Doctors don't know everything. And because they are human, they make mistakes, too. She says, "It was then I realized I had to start taking some responsibility for my own health care."

Even when a mammogram appears normal, all suspicious lumps should be biopsied for a definitive diagnosis. Fortunately, nearly 85 percent of all breast biopsies prove to be benign. But, based on the surgeon's comments, Malinda was pretty certain even before surgery that she was not as fortunate.

"Right away, the surgeon told us we could probably never have children," she remembers with pain. "My husband nearly fainted in the chair. The doctor tried to explain that the younger and healthier you are, the healthier your cancer is." In looking back, Malinda believes this was his way of telling them exactly how serious her condition was.

But the biggest shock for Malinda, and the information that continues to haunt her, was the doctor's opinion of how long her cancer had been growing. Because it appeared to be multiplying very rapidly, he speculated that Malinda probably hadn't had the tumor for more than two or three months. That means when she saw the first doctor, her disease was in its infancy. "Sometimes I think if I had just been a little more assertive with the first doctor, I might have saved myself some of the problems I'm going through now. Maybe if I had insisted on a mammogram that first visit, the cancer wouldn't have gotten into my lymph nodes." With inflammatory breast cancer, in all likelihood, lymph nodes would have been involved even if the cancer were found one month earlier.

Second guessing yourself after the fact is never very productive. But Malinda learned some important lessons that can benefit other women in similar situations:

- Early diagnosis and treatment are significant factors in breast cancer survival rates. If the cancer is localized and can be totally removed through surgery, the five-year survival rate is 96 percent. If the cancer has spread, the survival rate decreases.

- Second opinions make sense. Sometimes they save lives. If a woman is concerned about a lump or a change in her breasts, but her doctor wants to "just watch it," a second opinion is a wise decision.

The National Cancer Institute's goal for early detection of breast cancer is to increase to 80 percent the number of women ages 50 to 70 who have an annual physical examination and mammogram. One study showed that five-year survival was 22 percent better for cancers diagnosed by mammography compared with those diagnosed after a lump appeared.

Malinda had to go back to her first doctor for a pre-surgical examination. He asked if he could look at the breast and palpate it one more time. Her reply? "I said, 'Sure, I think you should so you'll recognize it the next time you see one like it.' He was very quiet through the whole incident. Of course, I never went back to him again."

Prostate Cancer

The weight loss and fatigue Lothair described when he was "running out of gas" were signs that his prostate tumor had already advanced to a noncurable stage. Prostate cancer is seldom curable once symptoms develop. At diagnosis, Lothair's cancer had already metastasized to his bones, severely limiting his treatment options.

At 65, Lothair fit the typical prostate cancer profile. More than 80 percent of all prostate cancers are detected in men over 65 years of age. But Lothair's diagnosis came without warning, before the now standard—but still somewhat controversial—PSA screening test.

In 1992, the National Cancer Institute doubled its funding for prostate cancer research based on the fact that incidence and mortality figures for prostate and breast cancer were roughly comparable. In 1993, 165,000 new cases of prostate cancer were predicted, with 35,000 deaths. In the same year, an estimated 183,000 cases of breast cancer were expected, with 46,300 deaths. Yet prostate cancer is receiving a fraction of the funding.

Part of the problem is the widespread notion that prostate cancer will eventually affect all men, that it is a harmless disease, and that most men will die of other causes before succumbing to prostate cancer. Such misinformation would explain the calm Lothair experienced upon hearing his diagnosis. But the size of his tumor and the bone metastases already present actually meant cure was impossible. Hormonal therapy was his only choice to slow the cancer's growth and reduce symptoms. After undergoing an orchiectomy (removal of the testicles), Lothair's body could no longer produce the male hormone testosterone, which helps prostate tumors thrive. His symptoms were immediately relieved. For many men, that relief sometimes lasts for years. But most likely, the tumor will return.

Researchers who encourage use of the prostate-specific antigen (PSA) claim Lothair's cancer would have been detected by this blood chemistry test during routine screening long before symptoms appeared. He then would have had more treatment options. Unfortunately, this was not the case.

Ovarian Cancer

Pain plagued Lou for months, causing her to double over in agony. When her ovary ruptured and she was rushed to the hospital for emergency surgery, the diagnosis of ovarian cancer took her completely by surprise.

Lou's diagnosis came at a time when few women knew much about the disease that currently strikes 22,000 each year, killing approximately 13,300. And it was long before Gilda Radner's public battle brought ovarian cancer into the limelight. At first, Lou's symptoms were vague, like those of many women— bloating and general feelings of stomach discomfort. Unfortunately, many women with early stage ovarian cancer have no symptoms. As a result, two-thirds of these women have advanced disease at the time of diagnosis.

As Lou's undiagnosed disease progressed, she complained of pain—first mild and later excruciating. Her gynecologist attributed the pain to an inflamed ovary. Only after the ovary ruptured was the cancer discovered. The surgeon labeled it slow growing and said he had removed as much as possible; no follow-up treatment was recommended. Ten years later, cancer appeared in Lou's liver. She was referred to an oncologist and started chemotherapy treatments.

By today's standards, Lou's original medical protocol sounds rudimentary, even bordering on malpractice. Perhaps it serves as an example of how far we've actually come in understanding how to diagnose and treat ovarian cancer. First, there seems to be a genetic predisposition to this cancer. Women with two close relatives (mother, sister, aunt, grandmother) who have had ovarian cancer have a 50 percent chance of developing the disease and should be watched closely.

Two recent advances make it easier to watch these women and find early cancers. The CA-125 blood test detects a cancer antigen shed into the blood by ovarian tumors. The test has proved valuable in gauging the success of treatment and monitoring high-risk women. But it is still not suited for widespread use, as it fails to detect nearly half of all early ovarian cancer.

Transvaginal ultrasound, in which a wandlike instrument is inserted into the vagina and scans the ovaries with sound waves, is a highly sensitive, accurate, and safe method of detecting enlargements that might be cancerous. If more studies confirm its success, transvaginal ultrasound could become a standard screening tool for women over 55 or younger women with a family history of ovarian cancer.

Taxol has been called the most promising cancer drug discovered in the last two decades. In clinical trials, doctors found that one-third of the women with advanced ovarian cancer who did not respond favorably to standard treatment showed a favorable response rate to taxol.

Colorectal Cancer

Colorectal cancer, which was once labeled "President Reagan's cancer," is the second most common cancer seen today (excluding common skin cancers). Approximately 150,000 new cases of colorectal cancer can be expected each year, with about 57,000 deaths. The incidence seems to be evenly divided between men and women.

John was already familiar with the warning signs of colorectal cancer—bleeding from the rectum, blood in the stool, or a change in bowel habits. People with a family history of colon cancer or with a history of polyps in the colon or rectum are at greater risk for developing this form of cancer. One authority believes 50 to 65 percent of bowel cancers develop from a pre-existing polyp.

A polyp of this type preceded John's diagnosis. After a frightening experience with bleeding from the rectum, John's doctor told him a polyp on his colon had ruptured. From that time on, both John and the doctor were on the lookout for additional colon problems.

Colon cancer can often be detected in its early stages by the stool blood slide test, flexible sigmoidoscopy and colonoscopy, and the digital rectal examination performed by the doctor. John's tumor, which was 10 inches up from the rectum, was found early during a routine screening.

Although public awareness of this cancer increased dramatically when former President Reagan had surgery, a national

American Cancer Society study found that most Americans over age 40 pay little attention to these organs and have few regular, thorough bowel exams. When colorectal cancer is detected and treated early, the five-year survival rate is 87 percent for colon cancer and 78 percent for rectal cancer. This compares with a survival rate of 47 percent and 38 percent, respectively, after the cancer has spread.

Another misconception is that anyone with colon or rectal cancer ends up with a permanent colostomy. To the contrary, one recent study showed that only 15 percent of patients whose rectal cancers were detected early required a colostomy. Colostomy after a colon cancer is rare.

As John learned with his colon cancer, time is of the essence. Surgery is still the best treatment. If the cancer is localized, often no follow-up treatment is necessary. If the cancer has spread to the lymph nodes, however, chemotherapy is frequently prescribed.

John talks about his experience: "One thing I've learned from our I CAN COPE classes is that you don't mess around with this stuff. When you find something that isn't the way it should be, find out about it." John took his own advice and is a healthy example of the benefits of early detection.

Clinical Trials

Whenever a new treatment method is discovered, extensive testing must be done before it can be offered to the general public. Although many people believe cancer research is done exclusively on laboratory rats, the ultimate cancer research is done on people. Whether a new biological therapy has just been approved after animal testing, or a new way of administering standard drugs has been found, the true test of treatment is whether it helps people with cancer.

In cancer research, studies using cancer patients are called clinical trials. These tests are carried out in phases, each having a different goal. The Phase I studies start immediately after the therapy is proven safe and active against cancer in animals. Human volunteers are then used to evaluate the safety or toxicity of the treatment. Although there is a small hope that the patient will benefit (1 to 3 percent), these trials are usually recommended for patients who have run out of options. These people with advanced cancer are, in effect, making a generous contribution to science by participating in the Phase I trials. The therapies they undergo are often dangerous, but every anticancer drug now used in therapy was initially part of a Phase I trial.

Phase II studies determine how effective the treatment is and against what specific types of cancer. For patients in Phase II trials, traditional treatment has usually failed or their cancer is not readily treatable.

Phase III studies compare the experimental drug to the standard treatment for cancer. Patients are randomly assigned to a treatment group, so whether a patient gets the new or the standard treatment is totally a matter of chance. But in a Phase III trial, one can expect to get a treatment comparable to the best treatment available. Phase III trials typically involve hundreds of patients and many hospitals and clinics across the country.

If you're asked to participate in a clinical trial, how should you make your decision? Grace Monaco, a member of a Food and Drug Administration Oncology Drug Advisory Committee and chair of the board of Candlelighters Childhood Cancer Foundation, advises that people should understand their own motives before participating in a trial. Can the treatment deliver what you're looking for? Just knowing the treatment could help isn't enough. Can you hope for cure or remission? Will it give relief or cause worse side effects? Physicians and patients need to use the same language and agree on definitions, which should be clearly spelled out in the informed consent form the patient must sign. Trials listed on the National Cancer Institute's Physician Data Query Program pass through additional peer review. That means the informed consent has been written with even more care, which is critical to the patient's welfare.

Irving Lerner, M.D., oncologist, agrees. "I'm totally in favor of clinical trials," he says. "But my primary obligation is to my patient. An individual interested in a Phase III clinical trail needs to be particularly well educated to ensure understanding of the good and bad ramifications. First, the patient doesn't want to lose the potential for success. Second, we hope this patient will ultimately help advance medical science . . . in that order, not the reverse."

To help sort out the options, a second opinion might be in order. The advice of a trusted oncologist not closely connected with the specific trial can give the patient a broader, more balanced view of the trial's advantages and disadvantages.

The majority of advances in cancer treatment over the past 20 years have come about because of clinical trials. Yet fewer than 5 percent of Americans who have cancer choose to participate. The National Cancer Institute would like to see those numbers go up. Any person interested in a clinical trial should discuss it thoroughly with an oncologist.

Cancer Research

Through both clinical trials and laboratory research, thousands of health care professionals across the United States are working to find a cure for cancer. Between the National Cancer Institute and the American Cancer Society, more than $3 billion are dedicated annually to cancer research in the United States. New therapies that make it to the third phase of clinical trials become experimental therapies.

Genetic engineering has devised new modes of diagnosis and treatment unimagined 15 years ago. Today, some biological response modifiers such as interferon and Interleuken-2 are already in clinical use. Many others are being tested in clinical trials.

Biological Response Modification

Conventional cancer treatment—surgery, radiation, or drug therapy—are harsh and unnatural. All three treatment forms impose unnatural forces on the patients in an attempt to eliminate the cancer. Much of the research currently being done focuses on a more natural approach—biological modifiers.

The term biological response modification means treating the cancer by using substances that occur naturally in the body, especially in the human immune system. The basis of any biological modifier is to take something from within, something that is already part of the body's defense system, and modify it so it can fight cancer cells.

Researchers now believe the immune system plays an important role in the development of cancer. One commonly held theory is that a properly functioning immune system is constantly rejecting malignant cells as they form in the body. If the immune system is not working properly, the malignant cells will continue to grow and eventually form a tumor.

Biological modifiers are not new to medicine. The smallpox vaccine is an example of a biological modifier. When people are vaccinated for smallpox, they are exposed to a small amount of cowpox, a disease very similar to smallpox. Once exposed, the human immune system strikes back by building strong antibodies to the cowpox. Those antibodies cross over and fight the smallpox. This same theory applies to both the polio and tetanus vaccines. To this day, the medical community still doesn't know how to cure these diseases, but they do know how to prevent them.

Scientists have been using this theory for more than 50 years in an attempt to give the body "just a touch" of cancer and force it to make enough protective antibodies to fight the disease.

Tumor Necrosis Factor

Tumor necrosis factor (TNF), an anti-tumor hormone, is the key player in a new technology that attempts to immunize patients against their own cancer. In a refinement of the "give the patient a little touch of cancer" theme, Steven Rosenberg, M.D., cancer researcher and chief of surgery at the National Cancer Institute, Bethesda, Maryland, was at the forefront. Doctors extracted tumor cells from two patients, inserted the gene that promotes production of TNF in the cells, and then let the genetically altered cells grow in a test tube for a week. The theory is that the "souped up" tumor cells, once reinjected in the patient, will kick the immune system into high gear to fight the specific malignancy.

Monoclonal Antibodies

Among the biological modifiers, many researchers are most excited about monoclonal antibodies. All cells make antibodies. When a cell becomes cancerous, its makeup often changes and a substance appears on the surface of the cell that is not found on normal cells. This foreign substance, called an antigen, must be present for a cancer cell to grow and divide. The goal of monoclonal antibody research is to develop an antibody that recognizes and attaches itself only to tumor cells, not to normal cells.

When animals are inoculated with a specific tumor antigen, they produce antibodies to that particular cancer. Researchers have developed a way to remove those antibodies from the animals and combine them with the patient's white blood cells. The patient is then injected with the mixture; the antibodies travel directly to the tumor cells.

About 200 of these antibodies have been produced in the laboratory so far. Although their major use today is to assist in diagnostic procedures, some are being used in early clinical trials with cancer patients. At Stanford University in California, patients with lymphoma have been treated with monoclonal antibodies. At the University of Minnesota, the antibodies are being tested in conjunction with bone marrow transplantation in people who have certain types of leukemia and lymphoma.

Monoclonal antibodies can serve several purposes, including the following:

- To kill cancer cells.

- To mark cancer cells for destruction. To be used most effectively, the monoclonals must be armed with a payload of "killer" drugs. The monoclonal then becomes a highly accurate delivery system that can zero in on a specific cancer site and destroy the malignancy without harming healthy tissue.

- To assist in diagnosis. A radioactive substance is attached to the monoclonal antibody. That substance goes directly to cancer cells, thus pinpointing the location of metastases previously undetected by other methods.

Stanley Order, M.D., an oncologist at Johns Hopkins University in Baltimore, believes monoclonals hold great promise in making selective chemotherapy possible. When attached to monoclonals, the chemicals can go directly to the cancer, providing the most efficient use of drugs with the least risk and discomfort to the patient.

Clinical trials are evaluating monoclonal antibodies by trying to determine how specific the antibody is against the target antigen on the tumor cell surface. As with all cancer therapy, side effects are a major concern, and the success of monoclonal antibodies will depend on how well the human system tolerates the foreign antibody.

Colony-Stimulating Factors

Although colony-stimulating factors (CSFs) are not directly effective against tumors, they do activate, regulate, and develop disease-fighting cells. By stimulating more rapid production of new blood cells, CSFs make chemotherapy patients less vulnerable to anemia and various infectious diseases. Once the fear of serious infection is out of the way, higher doses of chemotherapy can be used, theoretically leading to more complete remissions. Some CSFs are already in use in the clinical setting, while many more are still in the research stage.

Oncogenes

All parts of the body are made up of cells, and the cells are composed of genes. Each human cell is estimated to contain 50,000 to 100,000 genes. Genes define who we are—from where the ears are placed to the color of eyes or hair. But only about 100 of these genes regulate cell growth and division. Some genes promote cell growth. Others suppress cell growth. Both function normally during human growth and development. But genetic changes can turn normal to abnormal, controlled to uncontrolled, benign to malignant. Researchers now believe that cancer's multi-step process begins with an aberrant gene called an oncogene.

All human cells contain proto-oncogenes, genes that seem to play a vital role in manufacturing proteins that regulate cell growth. These proto-oncogenes are harmless—until a carcinogen comes along and, through some genetic mutation, changes the proto-oncogene into a cancer-causing oncogene. Once the oncogene is activated by a metabolic defect in the cell, it works with other genes to change a normal cell into a cancer cell. This metabolic defect, or DNA damage, may be inherited or may arise spontaneously after contact with a carcinogen.

Once the regulation of cell growth is impaired, the cell begins producing an abnormal protein that ultimately starts the growth of cancer. The cancer cells eventually accumulate and crowd out the normal cells, and a tumor is formed.

In laboratory experiments, the introduction of oncogenes into a tissue culture have repeatedly transformed benign cells into cancer cells. The next step, and the most exciting, would be determining what it is about the oncogene that makes cancer. With that knowledge, researchers could then work on ways to block the mechanism from ever coming into play, or perhaps do something to neutralize or counteract it. Such a solution may be a long way off—but it is possible. Approximately 50 oncogenes have been identified, and many oncologists believe that understanding these oncogenes and their protein products will eventually be the key that unlocks the mystery of cancer's origins.

Molecular biology truly came of age when the FDA approved the first DNA probe-based diagnostic test for chronic myeologenous leukemia based on the Philadelphia chromosome, a specific abnormality related to gene rearrangement. Similar probes are being developed to aid diagnosis of some leukemias and lymphomas, and they appear to be effective in recognizing gene rearrangements and mutations in many breast, ovary, and bladder cancers, as well as abnormalities in the colon and retina.

For the near future, discovering these genetic abnormalities will undoubtedly make it easier to detect cancer earlier, perhaps by identifying and isolating the abnormal protein produced. Such technology could help identify high-risk individuals (those who possess the suspect oncogene). Cancer in these individuals might be prevented by changes in lifestyle or perhaps by intercepting and halting the deadly message put out by the oncogene.

Lewis Thomas, M.D., retired chancellor of Memorial Sloan-Kettering Cancer Institute, predicted that we will be able to identify and cure all forms of cancer by the year 2000. The field of molecular biology—and specifically the identification of oncogenes—led him to make that prediction.

Quality of Life Issues

Clinical trials of new, experimental therapies often involve potential risk and unpleasant side effects. When do these negative side effects outweigh the survival gains associated with treatment?

In recent years, many professionals have begun asking that question. As a result, the NCI's Cancer Therapy Evaluation Program (CTEP) and the Division of Cancer Prevention and Control (DCPC) are now encouraging cooperative study groups to include quality of life (QOL) assessment as part of Phase III trials whenever feasible. In fact, the U.S. Food and Drug Administration recognizes benefit to QOL (as well as improved survival) as a basis for approval of new anticancer drugs.

Why the increased interest in this new QOL measurement? Because as cancer therapies became more toxic, small gains in survival were being achieved at significant physical and emotional cost to the patient. The goal of this research is to help physicians choose therapies that enhance rather than detract from a patient's overall well being.

By tuning in to a therapy's effect on quality of life, treatment decisions could be altered in three different ways. First, if two treatments yield similar results, a significantly better QOL could be the distinguishing factor between them. Second, a treatment may be considered effective therapeutically, but if QOL is diminished profoundly, the treatment might be deemed ineffective for general use. Third, a treatment that is less effective medically may be chosen because it is more successful in reducing symptoms, to the point where quality of life is enhanced.

A significant body of evidence also suggests that many interpersonal and psychological factors can influence the course and outcome for certain cancers and the quality of life for patients. Research on women with breast cancer has shown that group support not only improves quality of life, but physical health as well. In the early 1990s, the United States Legislature requested that the National Cancer Institute explore the impact on survival and quality of life from psychosocial counseling services as part of the medical care offered.

The Ultimate Cure—Prevention

All the advanced technology in the world will never equal the cure rate of prevention. After all, a cancer that never develops is 100 percent cured! Several known carcinogens and ways to avoid them have already been discussed. In an attempt to translate knowledge into the saving of human lives, the National Cancer Institute set a goal to cut the 1980 cancer mortality rate in half by the year 2000.

Only 50 percent of that reduction is expected to result from advanced technology. The rest will come through prevention. In the 1980s, the American Cancer Society launched one of the largest studies ever carried out in the United States on cancer prevention. This long-term study is examining the habits and exposures of more than one million Americans to learn how lifestyles and environmental factors affect the development of cancer.

Questions in the study focus on risks of certain drugs, foods, and various occupational exposures; low-tar and nicotine cigarettes; consumer products; and long-term exposure to low-level radiation. It is also examining the health effects associated with air and water pollution.

The goal of the study is to identify factors that increase a person's chances of developing cancer, those that carry little or no risk, and those that actually may help prevent cancer.

As knowledge of cancer and its causes broadens, it becomes clear that this complex group of diseases is influenced by both internal and external factors. Even if the body is predisposed to cancer's development, environmental factors appear to play a significant role in the development and growth of a cancer.

A popular myth holds that the individual is powerless against cancer. Today that myth is being challenged. The tools of prevention and early detection rest in the hands of every individual willing to use them.

Suggested Reading

To learn more about topics discussed in Chapter 1, the following reading material is recommended:

Altman, Roberta and Michael J. Sarg, M.D. *The Cancer Dictionary*. New York: Facts on File, 1992.

Brody, Jane E. *You Can Fight Cancer and Win*. New York: Quadrangel, The New York Times Book Co., 1977.

Dollinger, Malin, Ernest Rosenbaum, and Greg Cable. *Everyone's Guide to Cancer Therapy*. Kansas City: Andrews and McNeel, 1991. Comprehensive, clearly written, excellent material written by cancer experts.

Holleb, Arthur I., M.D., Editor, *The American Cancer Society Cancer Book: Prevention, Detection, Diagnosis, Treatment, Rehabilitation, Cure*. New York: Doubleday, 1986. This 650-page book includes topical essays by cancer experts. Gives addresses and phone numbers for all the Comprehensive Cancer Centers in the nation.

Laszlo, John, M.D., *Understanding Cancer*. New York: Harper & Row, 1987. Good information from a doctor who was a patient as well.

Morra, Marion, and Eve Potts. *Choices: Realistic Alternatives in Cancer Treatment*. New York: Avon Books, 1987 (revised edition). Written in question and answer format, comprehensively covers diagnosis, tests, treatments, and side effects.

Rosenbaum, Ernest H., and Isadora R. Rosenbaum. *A Comprehensive Guide for Cancer Patients and Their Families*. Palo Alto: Bull Publishing, 1980.

Ryder, Brent, Editor. *The Alpha Book on Cancer and Living*. Alameda, CA: Alpha Institute, 1993.

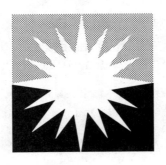

"I decided that if I was going

to take those drugs,

it would have to be

because <u>I wanted to</u>,

and because I believed

they were positive and

powerful allies of my body."

Neil A. Fiore, Ph.D.
<u>The Road Back to Health</u>

CHAPTER TWO

UNDERSTANDING CANCER TREATMENTS

When a child is diagnosed with a bacterial infection such as strep throat, there is one preferred way to treat it: penicillin. If the proper diagnosis has been made, there is little doubt that the treatment will be effective and the infection will be cleared up in a short time. Or when an adult is rushed to the hospital with an appendicitis attack, generally there will be little consultation before deciding to remove the appendix. Surgery cures the problem, and the patient goes home as good as new.

Cancer, an umbrella term that covers more than 150 different types of disease, is not diagnosed or treated so easily. Each cancer has its own special characteristics, and treatment choices vary based on the type of cancer and how early it is found. Before the discovery of penicillin, doctors couldn't identify a "right" or "wrong" way to treat bacterial infections either. Similarly, for many newly diagnosed cancer patients, no clear-cut "right" or "wrong" treatment choice exists. Instead, a specific treatment is tailored to a specific disease. Learning more about that specific disease requires thorough diagnostic testing.

Diagnostic Methods

A complete physical examination is the first step in diagnosing any illness. After taking a medical history, the doctor usually questions the patient regarding specific problems. Once problem areas are identified, the doctor focuses on specifics. A suspected diagnosis often determines the follow-up tests to be performed.

Blood Tests

Blood tests can be nonspecific or specific. Nonspecific tests call attention to abnormalities, giving doctors clues but not solutions. A specific diagnosis usually isn't based on these tests alone.

Cancers of blood cells (leukemias) are sometimes found with a simple blood test, and the diagnosis is confirmed by examining cells from the bone marrow. Multiple myeloma is also diagnosed through bone marrow analysis.

Specific tests are sometimes ordered if a doctor is looking for a tumor marker, a chemical sign of a specific cancer. A tumor marker is a biochemical indicator for the presence of a tumor. For instance, very high levels of a protein called carcinoembryonic antigen (CEA) strongly suggest tumor activity, specifically of the bowel, breast, or lung. An elevated CEA might prompt the doctor to follow up with more specific tests for these types of cancer.

Unfortunately, no tumor marker has been shown to be specific or sensitive enough to use in the detection of tumors in the general population, with the exception of the PSA test for prostate cancer. Currently, markers are most useful in tracking a cancer after treatment. Reappearance of a marker often signals a relapse.

For Bill, who remained in remission from testicular cancer for almost ten years, an elevated tumor marker was the first sign of recurrence. "At my checkup, the doctor looked over the records and said I could finally start coming at one-year intervals instead of every six months," Bill muses. "Two days later he called me back to say my AFP numbers were up." AFP (alpha-fetoprotein) is an oncofetal protein found in 20 to 70 percent of testicular tumor cases. The increase in AFP meant Bill's testicular cancer was probably active again.

"They put me through all the scans but couldn't find anything," Bill remembers. "I have so much scar tissue from previous surgeries, finding a new tumor became an almost impossible task." Even before pinpointing the exact location, the oncologist started Bill on chemotherapy. But after four months, Bill's AFP numbers were still unsatisfactory. More thorough imaging showed a tumor growing near Bill's left kidney. On Thanksgiving, he underwent surgery to have the kidney removed. After surgery, his AFP numbers plummeted back down to normal.

"Now I keep a log of those numbers," Bill says. "Some months they're up a little. Other months they're back down." He sometimes has second thoughts about keeping the log, wondering if it keeps him too focused on the illness. But Bill decided the numbers were too important to ignore.

Fluid and Stool Tests

Urinalysis, analyzing the urine's composition, can reveal abnormal protein levels or elevated white or red blood cells. For many years, the fecal occult blood test, a method of treating stool samples with a chemical to reveal blood, has been a standard diagnostic test. Some studies have cast doubt on the test, concluding that most cancers and a vast majority of precancerous lesions are missed. But despite the test's flaws, data from the University of Minnesota show decreased cancer mortality in persons conscientiously using this test. Most still consider it the best available means of inexpensively screening large populations for early colorectal cancer.

Scans and X-Rays

After the standard noninvasive tests, a doctor may decide to take a look inside the body by getting an image of suspicious areas. For many years, radiography (X-ray) was the only tool available. For doctors to see the digestive system on X-rays, a contrast medium such as barium was used. Barium fills the digestive tract to make it more distinct on X-ray film. Other substances such as dye or air can be injected into the system to help doctors see the kidney or other organs. Today doctors still use X-rays, but more exacting imaging techniques make diagnosis without exploratory surgery possible.

Computerized tomography scans (CT scans) produce images far superior to standard X-rays and allow doctors to see parts of the body the X-ray can't reach. The patient lies quietly on a table while a computer-directed X-ray tube revolves around, collecting thousands of pieces of information each second. The machine X-rays one thin layer of tissue after another, and a computer translates this information into cross-sectional pictures, which the doctor then studies. These pictures show a tumor's size, shape, and location more accurately than a standard x-ray.

For Debbie, the CT scan was the key diagnostic tool in discovering her brain tumor. Her medical history and previous tests pointed to a neurological problem, but the CT scan proved the existence of a tumor. Without that scan, Debbie probably would have endured a high-risk diagnostic procedure requiring injection of a dye along with conventional brain X-rays. A CT scan is not considered a high-risk procedure.

An even more sophisticated diagnostic tool that is commonly used is the magnetic resonance imaging (MRI) machine. The MRI scanner uses a powerful magnetic field to produce detailed images of internal organs without using radiation or X-rays. These three-dimensional images are nearly as detailed as the fine-line anatomical drawings in medical textbooks. Although MRI is used to scan all parts of the body, it is especially effective in viewing the brain and spine.

Nuclear medicine scans are another diagnostic tool that enables the doctor to diagnose diseases in the thyroid, bone, liver, gallbladder, or heart. The two most common nuclear scans used in cancer diagnosis are the liver scan and bone scan, two sites where metastases can occur. The patient swallows or is injected with a very small, safe amount of radioactive material, which then travels to the intended organ. Once there, the material emits gamma rays that are detected by a special camera. The pictures show the anatomical structure of the organ. In a liver scan, the isotopes settle in normal tissue so the image shows "cold spots" that could be cancerous areas. A bone scan is just the opposite; cancer cells in the bone take up the isotopes, and "hot spots" illuminate the skeleton. Hot spots can also result from bone injury or arthritis.

For Malinda, the bone scan was more than a diagnostic tool. Once the cancer had metastasized to her bones, scans monitored the growth of the cancer. Her doctors could determine the success of her treatment program by looking for changes in the scans. Malinda says, "The doctor said that if the cancer had gotten smaller or looked about the same, our treatment program could be considered successful. Sometimes I feel like I'm living from bone scan to bone scan."

Ultrasound creates images without X-rays by bouncing high-frequency sound waves off tissues and organs. These sound waves are then converted electronically into images. On the ultrasound picture, the technician can distinguish between a solid tumor and a cyst. The tumor looks darker on the picture because it has particles inside. A cyst filled with fluid appears lighter and hollow because fluid doesn't reflect ultrasound waves. A doctor cannot distinguish a malignant tumor from a benign tumor based on ultrasound alone. Transvaginal ultrasound and prostatic ultrasound are being investigated as potential diagnostic tools to increase early detection of ovarian and prostate cancers. Ultrasound has also been helpful in diagnosing tumors of the stomach, pancreas, kidney, and uterus.

Positron emission tomography (PET) is an imaging technique that identifies breast tumors most likely to respond to hormone therapy. It also locates hormone-receptive metastatic disease much earlier than previous tests were able to do. PET uses a radioactive tracer that binds to estrogen receptors in a woman's body. The technique actually "photographs" a tumor receptor and may prove to be most useful in targeting secondary tumors.

Endoscopy

When imaging isn't enough, doctors need to look inside the body cavities. This technique is called endoscopy. The doctor uses a flexible scope to see inside the lungs, stomach, colon, bladder, or other organs. The fiberoptic endoscope has a lighted tip for viewing. Flexible scopes use bundles of glass fibers that bend around all corners and enable the doctor to take pictures or sample cells from suspicious areas.

A fiberoptic bronchoscope examines lung passages and often makes it possible to diagnose lung cancer without surgery. A flexible gastroscope or colonoscope allows viewing of the entire colon and stomach. Tumors, cysts, polyps, and ulcers can be seen with the aid of these instruments, and tissue samples can be biopsied.

Biopsies

Once a tumor is found, the next step is to ascertain whether it is benign or malignant by looking at a small piece of tissue from the tumor itself under a microscope. This special test is called a biopsy. Sometimes the biopsy can be taken through the skin without doing surgery. But if the tumor is located deep inside the body, surgery is required.

In an incisional biopsy, the surgeon cuts into a portion of the tumor, whereas in an excisional biopsy the entire tumor is removed. In a needle biopsy, a very thin needle is directed into the tumor and a bit of tissue is withdrawn (fine needle aspiration). Tumors in the lung, liver, pancreas, and kidney can be diagnosed this way, and the procedure is most effective when done with a CT scanner directing the needle.

The biopsy is the most definitive and reliable method of diagnosing cancer. The pathologist who examines the tissue sample under the microscope plays a critical role in the diagnosis and subsequent treatment. If the pathologist finds a malignancy, the surgeon often asks for a second opinion from another pathologist. When the diagnosis is complicated, the case may be presented at a tumor conference where several doctors give opinions.

For Dave, the long road to diagnosis finally ended with a biopsy. Up until the surgeon found a small enlarged node under Dave's arm, doctors suspected everything from colon problems to gallbladder trouble. Hodgkin's disease is an uncommon malignancy and can only be diagnosed by looking at cells under a microscope. Once the pathologist identified the characteristic Reed-Sternberg cell, which is only present in a case of Hodgkin's Disease, Dave's wait for definitive answers was finally over.

Cancer Staging

The Reed-Sternberg cell that finally confirmed Dave's Hodgkin's disease diagnosis is a good example of how a tumor's appearance and behavior under the microscope reveal vital information. Generally, if tumor cells look much like the normal tissue cells from the same area, they are called well-differentiated. For instance, a pathologist could identify a well-differentiated breast cancer cell without being told the cell's origin because breast cells have a characteristic look. These tumors often are identified as "low-grade," meaning they are mature, well-differentiated, slow growing, and less aggressive.

Undifferentiated or poorly differentiated tumor cells don't necessarily look like the tissue of the organ where they originated. They are immature and don't resemble any specific tissue. Many times, the only way a pathologist knows the origin of these undifferentiated cells is by asking the surgeon. Poorly differentiated tumors tend to be more aggressive, grow faster, and spread earlier. These tumors are often identified as "high grade."

Flow cytometry, another way of examining cells, is a result of the blossoming field of DNA research. To date, the technology has been used most successfully in analyzing breast cancer cells. Since DNA is the genetic material responsible for normal growth and reproduction, an abnormal DNA content (DNA aneuploid) often suggests a poorly differentiated, aggressive cell. A tumor cell with a normal amount of DNA (DNA diploid) tends to be well differentiated, and the patient can expect a better prognosis.

Flow cytometry also analyzes the percent of breast cancer cells making new DNA, a term identified by the S-phase fraction. The percentage of tumor cells in the S-phase (tumor cells making new DNA) may be an indication of how rapidly a tumor is trying to grow. A high S-phase fraction suggests a rapidly growing cell and consequently a less favorable prognosis.

Because breast cancer seems to be associated with hormone levels, doctors also examine the estrogen and progesterone receptors of the biopsied breast cancer tissue. If the tumor contains a high level of estrogen or progesterone receptors, it is classified as positive, meaning the tumor is probably dependent on one or both of the hormones. In these cases, hormonal therapy becomes a treatment option. Malinda's tumor cells did not contain high levels of estrogen. Even though her diagnosis occurred before the DNA technology became available, her history and clinical exam suggested a rapidly growing, aggressive tumor.

How a Cancer is Staged

After collecting data from these tests, the doctor is able to identify the type of cancer, the size of the primary tumor, where it is located, if it has spread to nearby lymph nodes or to a distant site, and how aggressive the tumor seems to be. This is called staging. Knowing the exact stage of the cancer will determine the most desirable treatment program.

Most cancers are staged using a national classification system called TNM (tumor, node, metastasis). The letter T, with a number anywhere from 1 to 4 stands for the primary tumor, with the smallest number representing the smallest tumor. For instance, T1 would be a small tumor, while T4 would indicate a larger tumor that may have grown into surrounding tissue. The letter N, which also uses number 1 through 4, represents local lymph node involvement. A larger number means more nodes are involved, suggesting a more serious condition. The letter M, with a zero or plus sign, indicates whether there are distant metastases. A zero would mean the cancer had not spread to other parts of the body. A plus sign indicates the cancer is no longer confined to the primary site.

Once the TNM numbers are assigned, they are evaluated. Considered together, they determine one of four stages in the cancer's development. In general, a Stage I cancer is the most curable because it is localized with no lymph node involvement. On the opposite end, a Stage IV cancer has already metastasized to a distant location and is more advanced. Like everything else about cancer, staging is derived from the information available combined with the doctor's opinion. That opinion sometimes changes as more tests provide more information.

Dave's biopsy clearly showed Hodgkin's disease. The doctor then did further testing, including a bone marrow biopsy to identify how far the disease had spread. Results showed widespread involvement, including in the bone marrow, and Dave's disease was identified as Stage IVB, with the "B" signifying that symptoms were present.

When Debbie's tumor was located on the CT scan, her doctor seemed confident that it would be benign. Instead, it was malignant. When the surgeon performed the biopsy and examined the tumor with the naked eye, he thought it looked like a Grade 2 malignancy. Yet under the microscope, the pathologist identified a Grade 3 tumor. Why the difference?

Debbie had given her doctor a history filled with only minor symptoms, considering the size of her tumor. In the spectrum of malignancies, hers appeared to be a lazy tumor, one that moved slowly and took a long time to grow. This information allowed the doctor to be optimistic about the preliminary diagnosis.

Yet under the microscope, the pathologist observed fairly aggressive cells, and a Grade 3 label was applied to the tumor. In reality, the difference between a Grade 2 and Grade 3 brain tumor is far less discernible than between a Grade 1 and Grade 3. In Debbie's case, the fact that she complained of only minor symptoms, even though the tumor was quite large, was an equally important factor in determining the staging part of the diagnosis.

Clearly, a combination of physical examination, diagnostic tests, and biopsy with follow-up staging are all necessary before the proper diagnosis can be made. To some people, it seems like the tests go on forever. But thorough testing and tissue examination are essential for an accurate diagnosis.

If, at any stage of diagnosis, a person is uncomfortable and wants a second opinion, most doctors will be more than willing to arrange a consultation. In fact, the doctors themselves often seek out a second opinion, especially when there is a variation in the interpretation of test results.

Choosing a Treatment Plan

The key to successfully managing cancer is getting the best possible treatment as soon after diagnosis as possible. The make-up of the treatment team depends on the type of cancer. With her brain tumor, Debbie continued working with her neurologist. Both Debbie and Lothair ended up seeing a radiation oncologist because they were treated with radiation therapy. Some prostate cancer patients might only see a urologist. But most people are referred to a cancer specialist, called an oncologist.

The oncologist must take the accumulated test results into consideration before suggesting treatment options. What is the stage? Are lymph nodes involved? Any distant metastases? How do the cells behave—aggressively or nonaggressively? Are hormone receptors a factor? What are the benefits and risks of certain treatments based on personal factors—specifically age and other complicating medical problems. The patient plays a key role in this decision-making process. The health care team can suggest alternatives. But the final decision remains with the patient.

Sometimes even the doctors disagree on the most appropriate treatment. Many hospitals offering cancer treatment have tumor boards, a group of several specialists who meet to discuss particular cases and give opinions on the advantages and disadvantages of certain treatments. A pathologist might explain the biopsy results, the radiologist presents X-rays and scans, and the oncologist presents the overall case history. At the tumor conference, the oncologist gets input and ideas from a wide range of professionals.

While addressing an I CAN COPE class, William Scott, M.D., surgeon, Minneapolis, explained the complexity involved in deciding on an appropriate treatment. "In many cases, we can't say that there is only one right way to treat a person's cancer. Two people may be found to have cancer in the same location, but because of some small variation in cell type, presenting symptoms, or area of involvement, the recommended treatments will differ. This is different from most other diseases. For instance, if you have a gallbladder attack because of gallstones, the surgeon removes your gallbladder. One disease, one cure.

"This is not true of cancer, especially when the difference is whether or not lymph nodes are involved. If lymph nodes are found to be affected, the cancer is no longer confined to one specific area. This mandates that the treatment be far-reaching and more complex.

"Cancer is a multifactoral disease. You can't compare one person's cancer with another's. Each one is unique. Consequently, every treatment needs to be unique."

For years, doctors offered one of three treatment choices: surgery, radiation, or chemotherapy. Today, biological therapy has joined the ranks of accepted treatment modalities.

Surgery

Surgery remains the most successful treatment when the tumor is small and localized; more cures result from surgery than any other type of therapy. For years, surgeons took the one-stage approach. If a cancer was found during the diagnostic biopsy, the tumor was immediately removed while the patient was still under anesthesia. Now many people prefer the two-stage approach. The surgeon does only the biopsy. If the tumor is malignant, the patient and doctor plan follow-up treatment, which could include another operation.

Surgery to remove the primary lesion involves removing the visible cancer plus a large area of tissue surrounding the tumor. This is done in case there are cancer cells hiding in the apparently normal tissue near the tumor. The lymph glands near the organ are usually removed at the same time, since most tumors spread to the lymph nodes quite early. If the cancer has already spread to other parts of the body, the surgery could be used simply to relieve symptoms, or in combination with another form of treatment.

Debbie's brain tumor was a good candidate for surgery. Located in the front left lobe of the brain, it was accessible without risking serious damage to other parts of the brain. During the operation, the neurosurgeon removed all the cancerous material possible.

One might assume that malignant brain tumor tissue looks quite different from normal brain tissue and that distinguishing between the two types would not be difficult. Unfortunately, this is not the case. At the margins, the two look very much alike. Not wanting to remove any more than is absolutely necessary, the neurosurgeon must make a tough clinical decision: is this tumor or is this normal brain tissue? Debbie's surgeon stopped at a point where, in his clinical judgment, tumor was no longer visible. But, he surmised some tumor still remained that could not safely be removed.

If the surgeon had felt confident that the entire tumor had been removed in surgery, perhaps Debbie wouldn't have required follow-up treatment. This wasn't the case. Debbie's neurosurgeon recommended that she also receive radiation to the surgery site.

In the case of an early colon cancer, follow-up treatment after surgery often is unnecessary. John's case exemplified that fact. To make certain all cancerous tissue was removed, John's surgeon removed the cancerous tumor plus seven additional inches of the bowel. Fortunately, human beings have plenty of spare bowel and can get along quite comfortably when some is removed, so John's surgeon could safely take several inches on either side of the malignancy. An early cancer that has not spread to the outer bowel or the lymph nodes has an excellent surgical cure rate. Because John's cancer was found early, only surgery was required. If cancer is found in the lymph nodes, surgery is often followed by chemotherapy.

Lou wasn't yet 50 when she started experiencing abdominal pain. Her doctor didn't suspect ovarian cancer because the disease was rare in women under 50. This was the mid-60s when ovarian cancer wasn't well publicized. In time, she was rushed to the hospital with a ruptured ovary. The surgeon discovered the cancer and removed all he could see. But bits and pieces remained. He did not suggest follow-up treatment.

Six months later, the doctor did exploratory surgery and took tissue samples for examination. He found tissue and lymph nodes that contained cancer, again removed all that he could, and followed up with radiation treatments to the affected area. Today, although ovarian cancer is still difficult to cure, Lou probably would have received chemotherapy at the time of her first surgery. After several months of chemotherapy, the doctor might have then done "second-look" surgery to see if any cancer cells remained. Then Lou would have been closely monitored by using the CA125 blood serum test, an excellent tool for detecting a recurrence. Fortunately, Lou's cancer was slow-growing and didn't show signs of recurrence until ten years after her second surgery.

Radiation Therapy

Soon after the discovery of radiation and X-rays, scientists discovered that some cancer cells are more sensitive to the destructive effects of radiation than normal cells. Radiation therapy, sometimes called radiotherapy or irradiation, uses high-dose x-rays, electron beams, or radioactive isotopes to destroy cancer cells. Radiation may be used before surgery to shrink the size of a tumor, after surgery to slow the growth of any remaining cancer, or, when surgery isn't possible, to reduce symptoms and make the patient more comfortable. Methods of delivering radiation can be broadly divided between external and internal.

External Radiation Therapy

Before external radiation, a simulation is performed to locate the precise location of the tumor and mark the "radiation port"—the exact spot where the beam will be directed each day. Radiation treatments destroy some normal cells along with the cancer cells, but the radiation oncologist works out an optimal therapeutic ratio, with a goal of using maximum centigrays (cGys), or rads, to destroy tumor cells without destroying nearby normal cells. Only cells in the path of the beam are killed, so radiation therapy will not be effective against cancer cells that have broken away from the tumor and are circulating in the blood stream or have already settled in distant tissues.

Radiation therapy is the second most common form of cancer treatment. Estimates suggest that more than half of all cancer patients receive radiation sometime during their illness. When and how radiation is used depends on the size, location, and cell type of the tumor. Standard treatment runs five days a week for anywhere from one to several weeks.

One or more megavoltage machines may be used to produce the best results. The Cobalt 60, which became available in the 1950s, has radioactive substances inside. The linear accelerator, or betatron, creates its own radioactivity. Many of these machines use X-rays or electrons or a combination of both, called a mixed beam. The choice of treatment depends on the type and location of the cancer. An electron therapy beam might be better for treating cancers near the surface of the skin, while a 25-megavolt betatron X-ray beam might be used to treat cancers deeper in the body. The large machines, which some say "sound like a vacuum cleaner," are moved up and down or around so the radiation can be beamed at the tumor from different angles.

External radiation therapy may be used alone or in combination with other treatments. For instance, if a tumor can't be completely removed during surgery, the patient might be a candidate for a single high dose beam from a linear accelerator while still in the operating room. Another innovation combining surgery and radiation is stereotactic gamma knife radiosurgery. This technique is used for high-grade brain tumors or those that are completely or partially inaccessible with regular surgery. First, a CT or MRI scan is used to localize the target tumor. Then an individualized radiation dose is calculated by the computer. The patient wears a helmetlike device, and the gamma unit aims more than 200 sharply focused beams of Cobalt 60 photon radiation at the target. All beams intersect within the target tumor.

Because Debbie's neurosurgeon suspected that some residual cancer cells remained, Debbie started external radiation two weeks after surgery. She received treatment five days a week for six weeks, for a total of 30 treatments. When her first CT scan after completing radiation still showed signs of tumor, Debbie was concerned. But she was cautioned against jumping to conclusions. Generally, after finishing a course of radiation, it takes anywhere from two to three months, sometimes longer, to get the full effect of radiation and see total shrinkage of the tumor. Many people receiving radiation treatments are discouraged when they don't see and feel immediate results. Keep in mind that radiation remains in the system for a long time, and several weeks may elapse before the effects are noticeable.

In the case of advanced disease, when cure is not likely, radiation can still relieve symptoms and improve quality of life. Pressure, bleeding, and pain caused by the size of the tumor are reduced by shrinking it with radiation treatment.

By the time Lothair's prostate cancer was discovered, it had already metastasized to his bones. Removing the prostate wasn't an option, so doctors at the Mayo Clinic suggested removing the testicles, which would deprive tumor cells of testosterone and hopefully retard the tumor's growth.

Lothair consented to the surgery, and two days later, he felt wonderful. "I was up and around, continuously asking the doctors how I could possibly feel this good," he remembers. Lothair was hopeful that the cancer in his bones had also shrunk.

But when he returned to Mayo three months later, a bone scan revealed cancer in his rib cage. While he was participating in a four-month experimental drug program, the pain seemed better. Then his back and legs started to ache. More scans showed cancer in his spine. The doctors took Lothair off chemotherapy and started radiation. Before starting radiation treatments, Lothair's pain was almost unbearable. "I was on pain pills every four hours—sometimes even more often," he remembers. "I spent miserable hours lying on the sofa. I couldn't even get to the table for meals. You might say I was in bad, bad shape."

Lothair had a total of 20 radiation treatments, one per day, five days a week for four weeks. After that, he needed little or no pain medication. "Some days, I don't take even one pain pill. Actually, I am delighted with how I feel."

Radiation therapy took away the pain and improved Lothair's quality of life. His optimistic outlook and sense of humor returned. He even started joking with the radiation oncology staff, calling the technician "Cobalt Charlie." Trips to radiation therapy actually became enjoyable.

Bone metastases can be painful. Lothair learned that radiation can reduce that pain. Once a cancer has metastasized, a cure is sometimes difficult and control becomes the primary goal. External radiation therapy is an effective way of controlling painful symptoms.

Internal Radiation

By placing radioactive materials directly into or around the tumor site, very intense radiation can be given to a small area of the body. This internal radiation, sometimes called implant radiation, is often used for cancers of the head, neck, breast, uterus, thyroid, and prostate. It can be accomplished in several ways.

Interstitial radiation therapy places the radiation source directly into the tumor or surrounding structures. Most interstitial radiation is delivered by a removable implant. Tubes are surgically inserted into the tumor and a computerized treatment plan dictates the specific strength and certain time period of the "seed" to be delivered. When the dose is reached, usually after one to seven days, the tubes and seeds are removed. Sometimes a permanent implant is used, and the small radioactive seeds are left in the affected organ for several weeks or months, slowly delivering a specific dose of radiation to the tumor.

Intracavitary radiation places a container of radioactive material into a body cavity, most commonly the uterus. The material is left in place for 48 to 72 hours, then removed. This method allows very high doses of radiation while still protecting the surrounding tissue.

Chemotherapy

Chemotherapy is a broad term used to describe the use of cell-killing or cytotoxic drugs in the management of cancer. During World War II, almost by accident, doctors discovered that mustard gas seemed to shrink tumors associated with lymphoma. Scientists then began searching for more chemicals to control cancer. During the 1950s and 1960s they actually discovered a whole cluster of important new drugs. Experimentation proved that some cancers could be cured with drugs—specifically testicular cancer, leukemia, choriocarcinoma, and many cases of Hodgkin's disease.

Over the next few years, the discovery of new anticancer drugs slowed down considerably. Although as many as 50,000 new chemical products are analyzed annually, very few actually make it beyond the laboratories into the experimental drug testing programs. Today about 50 anticancer drugs are on the market and another dozen are available through clinical trials.

What makes chemotherapy unique? Drugs used in chemotherapy circulate throughout the body, reaching cancer cells that have broken away from solid tumors but are undetectable by normal diagnostic techniques. The disadvantage of this treatment is that these drugs are very potent, and they can affect normal as well as cancerous cells. For this reason, much of the research in chemotherapy today is aimed at finding ways to combine drugs most effectively so they can destroy cancer cells without harming normal cells. Most side effects of chemotherapy are caused by the damage done to normal cells. (For complete information on side effects, see Chapter 3, Managing the Effects of Illness and Treatment.)

Drug selection depends on many factors, including type of cancer, stage of cancer, reported experiences of other oncologists, and reports of research findings. Unfortunately, cancer treatment using chemotherapy is not an exact science. Two equally skilled oncologists might choose to treat the same patient with different chemical combinations administered on different time schedules. These differences exist because there is still no "right" or "wrong" way to treat some cancers. Both oncologists would no doubt be basing their choice of treatment on existing studies and other consultations that guide them in their decision making.

In the past, chemotherapy was used as a second line of defense, often not until after a recurrence. Current thinking seems to support the philosophy that "earlier is better," and many doctors are using adjuvant chemotherapy after successfully debulking a tumor through the use of surgery or radiation. The hope is that early chemotherapy will prevent or postpone recurrence by getting rid of undetectable micrometastases before they have a chance to grow.

Chemotherapy can also be used before surgery to reduce a tumor's size and make it more operable, and it is sometimes used to shrink nonoperable metastases that are already present. Although cure is the primary goal, more often chemotherapy is used to relieve pain and control tumor growth, enabling people to live longer and more comfortably than would have been possible without it.

Each chemotherapy program is unique and may include just one drug or a combination of drugs. When a combination of drugs is used, one drug might act on the cell when it is just starting to divide, while another strikes the cell when division is almost complete.

Two new methods of dosing and administering chemotherapy have developed in the past few years. The first follows the philosophy that if a little bit of a drug is good, a lot of the drug is better. Oncologists choose to give the drug in more intense doses over a shorter period of time. The second trend is to infuse the drugs continuously over a long period of time. This follows the philosophy that by maintaining effective levels in the blood, more cancer cells will be killed. The DNA technology that created colony-stimulating factors (CSFs), copies of natural body proteins that stimulate production of white blood cells to fight infection, makes intense, high-dose chemotherapy less risky. And introduction of more sophisticated drug delivery systems, especially ambulatory pumps, has made continuous infusion a relatively simple procedure.

Chemotherapy Delivery Systems

Pills, intravenous injections, or intravenous drips used to be the only way to receive chemotherapy. People with small and fragile veins suffered while health care professionals made multiple attempts to find a vein, especially after a few chemotherapy sessions. Today, several other options are available.

Venous Access Devices

Intravenous therapy with a venous access device involves placing a small, flexible, hollow tube, called a catheter, into a vein where it can be left for several months or more. The catheter extends into a vein in the neck, chest, or abdomen. Medications or other fluids are then given through the catheter directly into the vein.

A central venous catheter (indwelling or Hickman-type catheter) is a small, flexible, hollow tube with an injection cap on one end and a clamp. The end of the catheter is left outside the skin, while the flexible tube is thread through a vein to a point near the heart. These catheters have up to three inner lines, making it possible to give more than one medication or solution at the same time. Because the catheter tip is outside the body, the vein can be accessed without a needle stick through the skin. This means a portion of the catheter can be seen outside the chest, however, and it requires frequent care, even when not in use.

An implantable venous access device (called a port) has two major parts—a catheter and a portal. The portal is surgically placed under the skin, and the attached catheter threaded through a vein to a point just above the heart. The device is accessed by putting a needle through the skin and portal septum. The advantage is that the device is totally under the skin, so it cannot be seen. It requires minimal care, but a needle must be inserted through the skin each time the port is used.

Ambulatory Pumps

Internal or external ambulatory pumps now make it possible to receive medication by continuous or intermittent delivery. Continuous delivery permits a steady flow of medication. Intermittent delivery permits the infusion of a prescribed volume of drug over a specified period of time. This advance in technology makes chemotherapy more "user friendly" by giving the patient more choices. Use of ambulatory pumps makes it possible to receive chemotherapy somewhere other than a hospital or treatment center.

Chemotherapy: Personal Stories

Malinda wasn't thinking about a treatment program when she first came out of surgery. Instead, she was hopeful her biopsy would prove benign. Her hopes were soon shattered. She had barely awakened from anesthesia when she first heard the word chemotherapy. She remembers, "The surgeon held both my hands tightly and told me, 'You have cancer. I took as much as I could.'" But his best efforts weren't good enough. Malinda soon learned that 20 of 22 lymph nodes were also cancerous. Most oncologists would agree that starting chemotherapy as soon as possible was advisable. In fact, given the characteristics of Malinda's cancer, many oncologists might have prescribed chemotherapy before surgery to debulk the tumor, perhaps even a bone marrow transplant.

Follow-up tests soon showed that Malinda's cancer was not receptive to estrogen, hormone therapy was ruled out, and she was scheduled to start chemo as soon as she had recovered from surgery. Malinda's husband accompanied her to the first chemotherapy treatment, which was administered in the hospital. Nothing seemed to go right. The nurse was preoccupied and had trouble getting the IV going. She then was paged and left the room. She didn't return for almost an hour. This waiting added to Malinda's anxiety and fear. She says, "I still wasn't used to being sick, and lying in a hospital bed just reaffirmed that fact. My husband and I had a big fight, and he stomped out of the room. Having the surgery was enough. Needing chemotherapy a week later was more than I could handle. I just wasn't emotionally up to it yet."

Malinda was receiving a combination of three drugs: doxorubicin (Adriamycin), cyclophosphamide (Cytoxan), and 5-fluorouracil (5FU). After her first treatment, her mouth tasted of metal and she became nauseated despite religiously taking the antinausea pills. "I told the doctor I couldn't make it through another chemo treatment if it was going to be like that." At the next session, the doctor cut the chemotherapy dose down considerably, but she still got sick. Malinda had to experiment with several different antinausea medications before she found the right combination. Today, new drugs such as ondansetron help with the nausea and vomiting and make higher doses of chemotherapy more tolerable.

It's true that every person responds differently to medications. Malinda acted on her own intuition about what was happening in her body. Fortunately, she accurately reported all symptoms and side effects to her doctor, since health professionals administering medications rely on patients to let them know how the drug is being tolerated.

After several months of treatment, Malinda's blood counts dropped perilously low. The doctor stopped chemotherapy to give Malinda's blood time to return to normal. Malinda remembers being concerned: "By February, I was getting nervous about not having chemo. I think the doctor was getting nervous too." Instead of dreading the chemotherapy, Malinda was beginning to view it as her lifeline back to health. It became a friend, not an enemy.

Two months later, the doctor biopsied the bone marrow to make sure it was healthy and able to produce the needed blood cells. Assured that the bone marrow was adequate, he put Malinda back on chemotherapy but changed the schedule from monthly to weekly so the doses would be smaller and less harmful to her blood.

Malinda was beginning to gain confidence in her ability to act as her own advocate in getting the best medical treatment.

Before starting her new treatment program, she went to M.D. Anderson Cancer center in Houston, Texas, for a second opinion. "They ran me through the mill and agreed that because my blood was low, weekly treatments of Adriamycin would be appropriate. The only question they raised was about the wisdom of postponing my treatment for those months."

Malinda returned to Minneapolis confident she was following the correct path. Because her veins had been used extensively, finding a good vein for treatment was becoming a problem. At that point, she insisted on finding another way to receive chemotherapy. Her doctor recommended the Port-A-Cath (venous access device), which was implanted in a major vein near her breast and delivered the drugs directly into her bloodstream without repeated insertion of needles into superficial veins. Malinda used an ambulatory pump, which allowed her freedom to go about her daily activities while receiving treatment.

With this system in place, Malinda was comfortable and mobile during treatment and even started referring to it as "getting hooked up." She says, "That was a real breakthrough for me. First, I wouldn't have them sticking me with needles anymore. And second, I had the guts to stand up and ask for what I wanted. I had never talked to doctors that way before."

Malinda was on weekly Adriamycin from March until July. She would have a light dose for three weeks and a heavier dose on the fourth week. "I was still working and going in to get my drugs every Wednesday. Even though I didn't experience any real problems, I designated Wednesday my vacation day. I wasn't sick, but I thought I deserved the whole day off."

Adriamycin can't be taken indefinitely. Because of potential cumulative side effects, particularly involving the heart, people must stop the drug once they reach their maximum lifetime dose. Malinda was due to reach her limit in August; then she was to start on a new drug regimen consisting of cyclophosphamide, methotrexate, and fluorouracil (CMF). "That was fine with me. I was tolerating chemotherapy well, and it wasn't interfering with my life."

During this time, Malinda's husband had taken a new job in Louisiana and moved into temporary housing. Malinda felt secure with the medical treatment in Minnesota and chose to stay put. By the end of August, she was feeling stronger and began reconsidering the move. "If you feel you are handling your health okay, you feel like you can handle other things too. I even visited him in Louisiana and looked at houses. But I didn't want to do anything permanent yet."

Late in July, she began having backaches. She had just returned from Louisiana and had traveled alot during the summer. She blamed the backaches on the travel. A month passed and the pain wasn't getting any better. Her doctor ordered a bone scan. When someone from the hospital called and asked her to report back at 1 o'clock and bring a friend along, she knew what the news would be. The bone scan showed cancer in three different locations in her spine. The doctor wanted her to start radiation treatments the very next Monday.

"The first thing you do is panic all over again. The second time you hear you have cancer is different from the first time. The first time you're devastated. The second time you're disappointed. After all the hard work you've done, after how well you've been facing it, that it would have the nerve to come back." She was willing to start the radiation whenever necessary. But she was disappointed that the chemotherapy had not done for her what she hoped it would—take her into remission.

Bill was more fortunate. Chemotherapy for him lasted only four months. And it proved to be a very successful four months at that. Today, testicular cancer often can be cured with drug therapy. But the exact combination of drugs was not discovered until the late 1970s. Dr. Lerner describes his experience in treating testicular cancer: "When I started in training, testicular cancer was cured once in a while, but in the vast majority of cases, patients died of the disease and the treatment was pretty awful. Then Lawrence Einhorn, M.D., oncologist, a researcher at the University of Indiana, put together a package of already existing drugs and started trying them out in different combinations. When he combined them in a special way to treat testicular cancer, the cure rate was astronomical."

The importance of Dr. Einhorn's discovery is magnified by the fact that testicular cancer is primarily a disease of young men. Until his discovery, testicular cancer was the most common disease-caused death of men ages 20 to 30. Today the most common type of testicular cancer—seminoma—has a survival rate approaching 100 percent in cases detected and treated early.

When Bill's testicle was removed and cancer was found, the doctors decided to do a CT scan to see if more cancer was present. The scan showed a tumor the size of an orange growing near his liver and kidney. They asked him to report back to the hospital immediately for surgery. After the tumor was removed, Bill was given the option of receiving follow-up chemotherapy. The doctors made it clear that chemotherapy was not necessarily required at this point. Looking back, he says, "I guess I would have considered additional treatment if it hadn't been for my poor insurance coverage. Being self-employed and underinsured, most of my medical expenses at that point were coming out of my pocket."

Two months later, Bill experienced severe back pain. He thought he had been overworking the muscles damaged in surgery. He tried sitting in a hot tub of water, but the pain remained. When he returned to the doctor, another tumor was discovered in the same location as before. This time chemotherapy was not optional. If Bill was going to survive, it was required.

Once he was certain that treatment was necessary, Bill consulted several doctors. He wanted the best medical team he could find and settled on a group of three oncologists. Of the three, two agreed on the chemotherapy treatment to use. The third protested their plan, saying he would recommend a different approach to treatment. It was hard for Bill to make a choice and feel comfortable with his decision.

Bill's experience is an example of how treatment plans can vary from doctor to doctor. In this case, there was disagreement even within the same group. Bill put his confidence in the two doctors who agreed. They chose a therapy of three different drugs, which Bill was to receive in the hospital over a period of one week. He was then to have three weeks off, except for coming in every Monday for an additional dose of the third drug.

The dosage for anyone receiving chemotherapy is initially based on body weight. After the first treatment, dosages are adjusted according to the patient's response. The aftermath of Bill's first treatment turned out to be a harrowing experience. By the time Bill had completed his first week in the hospital, he was not only nauseated, but he was also unable to sleep. He went to his parents' farm to recuperate, but his body just didn't seem able to rebound. In fact, Bill became sicker.

Within a week, Bill was delusional, and he was rushed back to the hospital where he spent a week in intensive care. The doctors first thought the cancer had metastasized to his brain. In reality, Bill's body was simply reacting to the chemotherapy.

The use of chemotherapy has been likened to trying to rid your grass of dandelions without killing the whole lawn. When potent drugs are flowing through your veins, the intention is to kill cancer cells, but the healthy cells are always vulnerable. Bill was receiving three very potent drugs, and they were starting to attack his "lawn."

Within a week, Bill was back to normal, but it was a very difficult week for his parents. "Of the whole ordeal, that week was what broke my dad up. He was convinced I had a brain tumor," reported Bill. Once he had recovered, Bill's dosage was lowered. His final three treatments were uneventful, but tiring. During his hospital stays, a constant stream of visitors kept the nursing staff busy. "Sometimes I would have as many as 14 guys in my room. They turned the place into a zoo, but it was fun."

He was particularly fond of the nurse who gave him his first chemotherapy injection. She was young, about Bill's age, and very nervous. "She told me she didn't want to make me sick," he remembers. "I told her to look at the bright side. If she didn't do it, I might not be here at all. I think it was hard for her to care for me because we were so close in age. We got to be good friends, and I hope I made it easier for her to give chemo to other young people."

Bill's treatment schedule lasted four months. On New Year's Eve, he left the hospital for the last time. "Now, every New Year's Eve that comes around is a real celebration for me." When Bill had celebrated his third New Year's Eve without a recurrence, he started breathing a little easier. A young man, in the prime of life, had been put into a high-quality remission that would last more than ten years. Today, even after one recurrence and the removal of one kidney, Bill lives a healthy, active life. Without Dr. Einhorn's discovery, Bill's original cancer probably would have killed him. Fortunately for him, and for many other young men with testicular cancer, the right combination of drugs was found. Although the treatment was rigorous, uncomfortable, and not without its scary moments, Bill is a living chemotherapy success story.

Hormonal Therapy

Hormones are chemicals produced in the body that regulate the activity of certain cells or organs, In women, the ovaries secrete the hormone estrogen, which plays a large part in regulating the menstrual cycle. In men, the testes secrete a group of substances called androgens, the most familiar of which is testosterone. Both male and female hormones are responsible for development of sex characteristics.

Because hormones seem to play a role in the development of some cancers, specifically breast and prostate cancer, it stands to reason that hormone manipulation might have an effect on the rate of the cancer's growth. Hormonal therapy, sometimes lumped together with chemotherapy, treats cancer by inhibiting the production of natural hormones or by duplicating their effect. In patients whose cancer is receptive to hormones, or where the estrogen or androgen is actually encouraging that cancer's growth, hormonal therapy can slow the growth of the tumor. In some cases, it is completely stopped.

In the past, women were treated with male hormones and men with female hormones. More recently, both sexes are being treated with hormone antagonists—drugs that inhibit the production of male and female hormones. Probably the best-known example of a hormone antagonist is tamoxifen, which is used to treat breast cancer. In fact, because tamoxifen has proved so successful in reducing the risk of recurrent breast cancer, a nationwide five-year study is now being conducted to determine if tamoxifen should be used as a preventive drug by healthy women who are at high risk for breast cancer.

The growth of Malinda's cancer did not seem to be dependent on estrogen, so she wasn't a candidate for hormonal therapy. But the growth of Lothair's prostate cancer was slowed when he had surgery to remove the testicles, which deprived his system of further testosterone production. Hormonal therapy is often used in conjunction with radiation or chemotherapy, or both.

Bone Marrow Transplant

The most dramatic advance in the use of high-dose chemotherapy took place when the use of bone marrow transplant (BMT) evolved from experimental use to traditional therapy. In the early 1990s, BMT brought promise to between 7,000 and 10,000 people per year who previously would have had little hope for effective treatment.

Allogeneic transplants transfer marrow from one person to another. A dramatic and controversial example of allogeneic transplant took place in the United States in the early 1990s when a woman became pregnant in the hope that her new baby would eventually be the donor of life-saving marrow for an older daughter with leukemia. Her hopes were fulfilled; the baby girl proved to be a match for her older sister. When the child was old enough, a successful transplant was performed. Finding matched, but unrelated, individuals for allogeneic transplants, however, is much more difficult.

Autologous BMT, in which the patient is both the donor and the recipient of the bone marrow, is the more common type. This is used most frequently to treat patients with Hodgkin's disease or non-Hodgkin's lymphoma, but is also used to treat leukemia, aplastic anemia, and some solid tumors, such as breast and ovarian cancer.

The theory behind ABMT is straightforward and follows the "more is better" theory of chemotherapy. If a little chemotherapy is known to be somewhat effective, wouldn't 10 to 50 times the standard dose be even more effective? Many researchers say yes. But the problem in the past has always been the toxicity of such doses to the person's system, mainly the bone marrow, the site where new blood cells are produced.

In ABMT, approximately one pint of the patient's bone marrow is removed, or harvested, before the patient receives intensive chemotherapy. That marrow, which would otherwise have been destroyed by the chemo, is later returned to the body, theoretically, after all cancer cells have been eradicated by several days of high-dose chemotherapy or radiation. The entire procedure is somewhat dangerous and extremely costly, requiring up to six weeks of hospitalization.

A modification of this procedure is called a peripheral stem-cell transplant, where stem cells (the special "parent" cells found in greater number in the bone marrow) are collected from the patient's own blood supply and then reinfused after high-dose chemotherapy. Recovery time is generally about a week less than for ABMT. The advantage of this procedure is that the patient requires no hospitalization or general anesthesia for the harvesting, and the harvesting of cancer cells along with stem cells is less likely.

When Dave's Hodgkin's disease recurred six months after he completed chemotherapy, his oncologist was not optimistic about the potential success of additional chemotherapy.

"He told us I could have more chemo, but it was quite possible the cancer would just recur again," Dave remembers. And Dave got a second shock at the same time. "He told us that BMTs were a specialty, and I would need to see a new doctor. He referred us to a university setting."

The recurrence of cancer, a dangerous new procedure, and a new doctor, all at the same time, seemed more than Dave could handle. He admits to being scared at that point. He had developed a trusting relationship with his oncologist over the previous two years; now he seemed to be dismissing Dave with a wave of the hand at a most vulnerable moment. Dave understood chemotherapy and was used to it; but bone marrow transplant was a mystery. He was walking into uncharted territory. And that frightened him.

Dave and Loretta soon regrouped and took on the challenge of finding the best medical care possible. The university setting proved unsatisfactory for them, since Dave would have to be part of a randomized clinical trial and couldn't be assured he would receive the bone marrow transplant. They chose instead to go to a large private hospital with a BMT unit. Dave's new clinical oncologist specialized in bone marrow transplant, and Dave instantly felt comfortable about making that decision. Loretta remembers watching the rapport develop between Dave and the young doctor. "Everything about the office environment was inviting," she says. "We felt well taken care of from the moment we walked in the door for the first consultation."

Before going in for the transplant, Dave spent several weekends in the hospital receiving chemotherapy in an attempt to eradicate as many cancer cells as possible before harvesting his marrow. "I remember that as the worst," Dave says. "I don't know if it was the chemicals making me crazy, or just the anticipation. I wanted to get the preliminaries over with and get in there for the transplant."

"I love a parade," Dave wrote in his journal remembering his first day in the hospital. And what a parade it was. Once in his room, Dave was greeted by his day nurse, a resident, a medical student, a dietitian, the lab tech team to draw blood, two IV team nurses, his oncologist and partner, the transplant coordinator, the evening nurse, med tech for an in-room electrocardiogram, the infectious disease specialist, and the night nurse. Including his wife and children, Dave counted 19 people involved in getting his therapy program going that day. He was now equipped with a high-tech venous access device with a triple lumen catheter, meaning he could be receiving three different solutions at one time. At about 2 a.m. that first day in the hospital, Dave's night nurse, Mimi, finally got the first chemo running into his system. "The night went slow," Dave concluded. "Just Mimi and me and not much sleep, but lots of monitoring of vital signs."

Biological Therapy

Biological therapy, which uses the body's own immune system to fight cancer, is the newest type of treatment and appears to offer promise for the future. Up until very recently, biotherapy was limited to study in medical laboratories. Today, several types of biotherapy are not only being clinically tested but are commonly used.

Most scientists believe that cancer results when the human immune system fails to operate correctly. Cancer cells probably occur in our bodies with some frequency, and most of us repel them without ever being aware of their existence. Some people, however, do not have a strong enough immune system to kill off the abnormal cells, and the cancer grows. Biological therapy is designed to stimulate the body's natural defenses to control the growth of the cancer.

Interferons (IFN)

Interferon, discovered in 1957, has been shown to stop viruses from reproducing and can heighten a patient's immune response. It is a protein the body produces naturally in response to viral infections and seems to actively recruit those types of immune cells that can best destroy some forms of cancer. Although interferon was once hailed as the potential cancer panacea, ongoing research trials have proved disappointing. Interferon-alpha does cause tumors to shrink 15 to 20 percent of the time in patients with kidney cancer, and some leukemias also respond well. Interferon seems to work best against diseases thought to be caused by a virus.

Perhaps interferon's real value was the role it played in promoting research into other biologic response modifiers. Interferon itself will undoubtedly prove most beneficial when used in combination with other cancer-fighting agents.

Interleukins

Vincent T. DeVita, Jr., M.D., of Memorial Sloan-Kettering Cancer Center and former National Cancer Institute director, called Interleukin-2 "the most interesting and exciting biological therapy we've seen so far." A few years later, the Food and Drug Administration (FDA) approved IL-2 for treatment of metastatic renal cell carcinoma (kidney cancer), where studies showed a response rate of 20 to 25 percent. Using IL-2 to treat advanced malignant melanoma has a similar response rate.

In a process called adoptive immunotherapy, IL-2, which enhances immune function, is cultured in a test tube with the patient's own white blood cells (lymphocytes). The cultured cells are then returned to the body along with additional doses of straight IL-2. Some researchers believe this modification results in a more effective treatment. Research and clinical trials continue on newer forms of interleukin.

Colony-Stimulating Factors (CSFs)

Colony-stimulating factors, which stimulate the growth of blood cells in the bone marrow, are hormone-like substances naturally produced by various cells in the body. Although this form of biological therapy is not directly effective against tumors, it does play a major role in enhancing treatment success. Intensive chemotherapy dramatically reduces the number of white blood cells, particularly neutrophils, that fight infection, making the patient a ripe candidate for any number of infectious diseases. When this occurs, the CSF drug can stimulate the production of the neutrophils.

The use of high-dose chemotherapy, particularly for bone marrow transplants, would be far more dangerous if it weren't for the boosted infection-fighting power provided by the family of CSFs. Thanks to increased research in recombinant DNA, CSFs can now be manufactured in large quantities using techniques of genetic engineering. And because of this, patients like Dave, banking on bone marrow transplants to put them in high-quality remission, are likely to have fewer and less severe infections.

Questionable Methods of Cancer Treatment

Laetrile. Krebiozen. Hoxsey's Herbal Tonic Treatment. Do any of these names sound familiar? Each one received significant press coverage in its day as the "sure cure" for cancer. In fact, their claims to cure cancer were totally fraudulent. None fulfilled the promise of being the "sure cure."

The American Cancer Society defines questionable methods as "lifestyle practices, clinical tests, or therapeutic modalities that are promoted for general use for the prevention, diagnosis, or treatment of cancer and which are, on the basis of careful review by scientists and/or clinicians, not deemed to have real evidence of value." Hoping for a miracle, many people fall victim to these worthless and fraudulent "cures" each year, and both their health and their pocketbooks suffer. It is estimated that some $2 billion to $3 billion is spent each year on questionable methods. And this money is often spent by intelligent, well-educated people. How can this be?

Fear, coupled with a certain distrust of the high-tech medical world, might be the answer. People who trust regular medicine are the least likely to use questionable treatments. On the other hand, people who feel negatively about their experiences with physicians are more likely to use unorthodox methods, as are people who believe that disease (especially their type of cancer) is caused mainly by poor nutrition, stress, and worry. Chemotherapy and radiation treatments can be unpleasant. When someone offers a miracle cure that is painless and quick, common sense is often overcome by a desire to believe that these conventional therapies are useless or more harmful than helpful.

Dangers of Questionable Methods

The strongest selling point for many of these methods often is that the patient has "nothing to lose." In fact, the patient has a great deal to lose.

Delayed treatment. Early diagnosis and prompt treatment are the keys to success in cancer treatment. Any delay caused by dabbling in unorthodox treatments lessens the chances for a cure.

Decreased quality of life. In a study comparing patients using conventional therapy with patients given unproven vaccines, a vegetarian diet, and coffee enemas, average survival time proved to be about equal. But the group on conventional therapy reported less pain and greater appetite, important quality-of-life issues for many cancer patients.

Serious physical harm. Questionable methods are not harmless. Laetrile, a substance prepared from apricot pits, was the "sure cure" of the 1970s. But Laetrile is 6 percent cyanide by weight, so ingesting a Laetrile capsule was actually a dangerous proposition. If the person's stomach contained foods that could cause the Laetrile to break down and release the cyanide, the result could be disastrous.

Financial harm. Few situations are sadder than watching a family spend its last valuable months and their last available cash on a fraudulent, useless treatment.

Characteristics of Questionable Methods

What can a person watch out for when assessing a questionable cancer treatment? Using Laetrile as an example, some general characteristics of questionable methods surface:

They Claim to Be Panaceas for All Cancers

Laetrile was used to treat all cancers, with preposterously high, though unproved, success rates. Supposedly, Laetrile worked on all forms of cancer, even though every cancer is unique and responds to different treatments. A drug that is very effective against leukemia may have little or no success in breast cancer treatment. Any treatment method that is said to be equally successful against all cancers should be questioned.

They Are Overly Simplistic

Questionable methods offer a simplistic concept of cancer and a simplistic concept of cancer treatment. The theory behind Laetrile was that every cancer was caused by a vitamin deficiency, an unsophisticated and naive generalization about a very complex disease. Today's popular questionable therapies are aimed at demystifying and simplifying medicine, perhaps as a revolt against technological, heroic medicine. People want a simplistic explanation for why cancer develops, and then rely on self-care and "natural" cures.

Vitamins figure into many questionable treatment plans. For instance, Laetrile was erroneously referred to as vitamin B_{17}. Unfortunately, the production and sale of vitamins is difficult to monitor. Although the FDA has strict standards for allowing new drugs on the market, control over vitamins is less stringent. Since vitamins are classified as food, they are far easier to get to market than drugs. The vitamin industry is very powerful in this country. By calling Laetrile a vitamin and cancer a vitamin-deficiency disease, the promoters of this drug created a very simple notion out of a complicated subject.

They Claim to Be Harmless, Painless, and Nontoxic

A sure way to attract someone with cancer is to offer a treatment that is painless and nontoxic. Conventional treatment has well-known side effects. A safe, nontoxic treatment probably would sound very appealing to someone who has just gone through several months of chemotherapy. In most cases, if the treatment sounds safe and easy, it's probably not for real. In fact, when substances are being ingested or injected, the treatment method could be quite harmful.

They Make Popular News Stories

Any cancer treatment introduced through the mass media as opposed to a respected medical journal should immediately be questioned. Because promoters of these methods do not have sufficient scientific data, they are unable to publish in scientific journals. They must instead depend upon the mass media—newspapers, magazines, and television—to pick up their stories and circulate them. Sometimes, these promoters publish their own pseudoscientific literature and claim it is scientific.

Anyone can claim to be a cancer treatment expert. To find out whether someone is truly qualified to treat cancer, a number of directories are available. These include the Directory of Medical Specialists, and the directories of the American Federation of Clinical Oncologic Societies, the American Association for Cancer Research, and the American Society of Clinical Oncology. The people listed in these directories are recognized as having special training and experience in cancer research and treatment. Any public or medical library can help you locate these directories.

The success of questionable therapies is almost always reported in the form of testimonials rather than controlled studies. Reports in scientific journals of long-term, controlled studies using mice to test a new cancer drug make for boring reading. Certainly it's more interesting and more moving to watch a beautiful young child on television whose parents are condemning the drugs that made the child sick and singing the praises of some special diet that has supposedly cured him.

Testimonials aired on national television are powerfully persuasive, even though the claims made this way can be totally false. It's no wonder that people still travel across the United States border to Mexico for the very expensive "privilege" of having their cancer cured with a new metabolic, "natural therapy of cellular detoxification and restoration." The wise consumer knows there is no such thing as cellular detoxification and restoration—and that these treatments are neither natural nor safe.

Promoters of Questionable Methods Claim Freedom of Choice

In a climate where the medical monopoly or cancer establishment is sometimes distrusted, promoters know that appealing to people's freedom of choice can be a successful selling tactic. One of the most sensitive areas is who has the "right" to decide on the best treatment for a minor—the parents or the medical specialists? Promoters of questionable therapies will say the parents should be able to choose their product over conventional therapy. The medical specialists say, and with volumes of evidence to support their conclusion, that to use a questionable method instead of conventional therapy represents a threat to the child's life. Instead of demanding accountability on the part of slick promoters, "health freedom" advocates place the burden of responsibility for making the wrong health-care choices on the patients and their loved ones.

Questionable Methods Versus Complementary Methods

When do complementary activities such as nutritional therapy, relaxation therapy, yoga, or effective support systems become questionable? When they promise a cure. Used in conjunction with standard therapies, these techniques often help decrease anxiety, depression, and pain. Individual and group support can have a positive effect on quality of life and overall attitude. But dietary programs and the right attitude alone won't cure cancer, and anyone making such claims is turning these helpful therapies into guilt-producing, questionable treatment methods.

Rejecting Questionable Methods Takes Courage

Promoters of unproven methods should not have the freedom to misrepresent facts and sell worthless cures to a vulnerable public. Allowing these promoters to operate without restrictions is like giving them a license to steal. With all the evidence accumulated against them, why do these promoters continue to thrive? Why do intelligent, affluent, rational people place their lives in the hands of an unskilled promoter whose "cure" lacks a single shred of scientific evidence supporting its value?

Dr. Irving Lerner has an interesting philosophy about that question. Based on years of experience with cancer patients, he believes it boils down to how much courage the person possesses. He says, "I enjoy being in this field because it gives me an opportunity to witness a great deal of courage in a great many people. Facing the fear, the harsh reality of a bad disease and a bad treatment, and often a poor outlook—all that takes an immense amount of courage."

Most people find within themselves the courage necessary to face cancer head on and make difficult choices regarding treatment and rehabilitation. For people whose fears are irrational and out of control, however, courage does not come easily. "People who do not have that courage tend to retreat emotionally," Dr. Lerner continued. "They resort to an earlier way of doing things. It is less intellectual, more emotional, more childish." He labels such methods as the "Mommy's kiss approach." When children are hurt, Mommy's first response is to kiss it and make it better. It's simple. It's safe. It's comfortable. It's warm. And it always works. But does it really?

Anyone with an advanced cancer who is facing uncomfortable treatment and uncertain results will undoubtedly be encouraged by a well-meaning relative or friend who suggests a questionable method. This creates an intense struggle between emotion and intellect. When considering any unknown method, the wise patient asks the following questions:

Guide to Questionable Therapies

- Is this treatment based on an unproved theory?

- Do treatments require unusual nutritional supplements?

- Is the treatment billed as harmless, painless, and nontoxic?

- Has the treatment been through clinical trials? Are claims backed up with controlled studies published in respected medical journals, or just through pamphlets or the mass media?

- Could the claims be true simply through the power of suggestion?

- Are the promoters recognized cancer treatment experts?

- Do the promoters attack the "medical establishment?"

- Do the promoters demand "freedom of choice" without accountability?

Despite the logic disputing these therapies, questionable methods have proven to be powerfully seductive and persistent through the years. Desperate people are easily persuaded by testimonials from people who have firsthand experience with cancer. When someone looks you in the eye and says, "This new and wonderful therapy cured me of my cancer. Look, I'm living proof," the tendency is to believe him or her. Before you do, however, consider the alternatives. Perhaps a proven therapy put that person in remission. Perhaps the cancer is progressing but is erroneously being reported as cured. Perhaps the person never had cancer at all. In even rarer cases, a spontaneous remission might have occurred. The wise cancer consumer needs to review critically the principles and concepts on which questionable methods are based.

The child with the strep infection will get better with Mommy's kiss, but only if it comes after a shot of penicillin. Unfortunately, such a simple treatment is not yet available for the person with cancer. New discoveries are being made every day that make cancer treatment more promising, and yet more confusing. Difficult choices must be made. But if you are willing to invest the time necessary to learn about your individual cancer and consult with one or more respected oncologists, your chances of making the right choice are excellent.

Suggested Reading

To learn more about topics discussed in Chapter 2, the following reading material is recommended:

Berger, K., and J. Bostwick. *A Woman's Decision: Breast Care, Treatment, and Reconstruction.* New York: Ballantine Books, 1985. Discusses options for breast cancer treatment and reconstructive surgery.

Brinker, Nancy. *The Race Is Run One Step at a Time: My Personal Struggle and Everywoman's Guide to Taking Charge of Breast Cancer.* New York: Simon and Schuster, 1990.

Kauffman, D.G., *Surviving Cancer: A Practical Guide For Those Fighting to Win.* Washington, D.C.: Acropolis Books, 1989. Excellent book, concretely written by a cancer survivor.

Love, Susan, with Karen Lindsey. *Dr. Susan Love's Breast Book.* Reading, Mass.: Addison-Wesley, 1990. Comprehensive guide to everything you could want to know about women's breasts and breast cancer.

Reich, Paul R., M.D. *The Facts About Chemotherapy: The Essential Guide for Cancer Patients and Their Families.* Consumer Reports Books, 1991.

United States Pharmacopeial Convention, Inc. *Advice for the Patient: Drug Information in Lay Language.* Mack Printing Company, 1990. Information on drug uses and precautions.

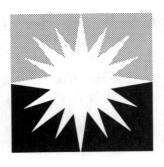

"It was day number one

in my new life

as a human being

with cancer.

And since it was incurable,

there would never be a morning

when I would wake up

without it."

Paul Tsongas
<u>Heading Home</u>

CHAPTER THREE

MANAGING THE EFFECTS OF ILLNESS AND TREATMENT

It begins with nausea and vomiting. Foods that only a month ago appealed to you now make you sick. You can't seem to drag yourself out of bed in the morning, and an afternoon nap can come none too soon. In the course of a single day, your mood can jump from euphoric and optimistic to negative and depressed. As time goes on, you gain more weight than you would like. Your feet and ankles swell, and you feel unattractive and obvious. Constipation becomes a problem. No matter what you eat or drink, your body seems to rebel. Insomnia has you staring at your digital clock at 2:45 a.m., your eyes wide open. You worry about the future. You fear pain. What is this person experiencing? Pregnancy.

Pregnancy and a cancer diagnosis are both major life changes, and this pregnant woman and the person going through cancer treatment are actually similar in many ways. Both experience physical changes as their bodies adjust to a new foreign substance. Both experience emotional upheaval as they struggle to adapt to a new body image and changed intimate relationships. Both experience a certain amount of anxiety not knowing exactly what lies ahead.

And just as every woman is different when going through pregnancy, each person responds to cancer treatment in an individual way. Some women never miss a beat from the moment of conception to the day of delivery. They claim pregnancy is the best thing that ever happened to them, and they have more energy and feel healthier than ever before. Others literally fall apart and experience all the symptoms mentioned earlier.

Reactions of people going through cancer treatment also vary. Unfortunately, the negative side effects of cancer treatment get the most publicity. A common cancer witticism, heard as often from doctors as from patients, is "the treatment is worse than the disease." For some people, treatment can result in uncomfortable side effects. But not all people will experience those side effects. Many are surprised to find that radiation is completely painless and chemotherapy brings on only minimal discomfort. This pleasant surprise sometimes causes anxiety. Many people believe that the therapy must have unpleasant side effects if it is to be successful. This is not true.

What accounts for such differences? There is no clear answer for that question. Certainly the type of cancer, the combination of drugs used, and the dosages all play a part. But another important factor, one that is totally controlled by the person with cancer, is nutrition.

The Importance of Good Nutrition

A pregnant woman needs to eat properly to assure optimum development of her baby. The fetus is creating millions of new cells daily. Those new cells will not develop normally unless the mother eats the right foods every day. Likewise, people with cancer, especially those undergoing treatment, require adequate nutrition and calories. Good nutrition results in many positive side effects, including:

- Researchers have found that people who eat well during treatment are better able to withstand the side effects of treatment. They may even be able to withstand a higher dose of some treatments.

- Good nutrition gives energy. Just as an automobile is powered by fuel, we are powered by proper diet. Going through treatment requires extra strength. A balanced diet prevents body tissues from breaking down and helps rebuild normal tissue affected by treatment.

- People with cancer who practice good eating habits have fewer infections and are able to be up and about more.

- Inadequate diet forces the body to use stored-up protein and fat for energy. With good nutrition, those nutrients can be used for a far more important job—rebuilding cells that have been damaged.

Nutritional Basics During Treatment

In addition to choosing foods from all four of the main food groups (dairy, protein, cereals and grains, and fruits and vegetables), people undergoing treatment usually need to pay special attention to protein and total caloric intake.

Protein

Protein is one of the chief components of all cells. It is necessary for the maintenance, growth, and repair of tissues. Additional protein is required during treatment because healthy cells are constantly being destroyed and need rebuilding.

How much protein is necessary? During illness, treatment, and recovery, a person requires between 75 and 100 grams of protein daily.

Milk products are a good source of protein. Two glasses of milk supply 16 grams of protein. People who do not enjoy milk can substitute cheese, ice cream, pudding, yogurt, and creamed soups. If digesting milk is a problem, lactase (an enzyme that breaks down the milk) can be added to ease digestion.

Until you are certain your protein intake is adequate, it is a good idea to keep a record of the grams of protein you eat each day. That way it is easy to see at the end of the day whether or not you are meeting the 75- to 100-gram requirement. If not, there are several easy ways to increase protein intake without greatly increasing your quantity of food.

Foods High in Protein

1 c. yogurt	10 gm.
1/4 c. cottage cheese	8 gm.
1 c. milk	8 gm.
1/2 c. baked beans	8 gm.
1 oz. meat, fish, poultry, cheese	7 gm.
1 egg	6 gm.
1/4 c. dry skim milk powder	6 gm.
3/4 c. split pea or cream soup	5 gm.
1/2 c. pudding	4 gm.
1 tbsp. peanut butter	4 gm.
1 c. frozen yogurt	4 gm.

Hints for Increased Protein Intake

- High-protein milk is the perfect solution for those who need good things in small packages. It is made by adding 1 cup dried skim milk to 1 quart of fluid whole milk. One cup of high-protein milk provides twice as much protein as a cup of regular milk. This high-protein milk can be substituted any-where you would normally use milk. It can be used in cream soups, on hot cereal, or in custards, puddings, and tapioca. High-protein milk is excellent in creamed tuna fish or for hot cocoa. If you don't need the extra calories but do need the extra protein, high-protein milk can be made with 1 quart skim milk instead of whole milk.

- Add small pieces of meat or cheese to salads, casseroles, or soups. For example, if you add some chicken to a can of cream of mushroom soup thickened with milk, your protein intake jumps dramatically.

- Cheese is concentrated protein. One ounce, or one slice of American cheese, contains 7 grams of protein. Cheese is easily added to soups or sauces. A cheese sauce on hot vegetables is especially good because it is both soothing to the mouth and gives additional protein.

- Peanut butter is also a concentrated protein. Spreading peanut butter on toast or on celery is a good idea.

- Dried skim milk powder can be added to many foods. One-third cup (about 5 tablespoons) of dried skim milk powder gives you 8 grams of protein. It can easily be added to hot or cold cereals, scrambled eggs, soups, and gravies. When making meat loaf or meatballs, the powder can be added right along with the bread or cracker crumbs. It can also be added to muffin or cake batters before baking.

Counting Calories

Calories equal energy. The number of calories you require daily is based on your age, sex, health, activity, and size. Generally, men require more calories than women. When people are undergoing chemotherapy or radiation, their calorie needs are higher than normal because damaged body tissues must be repaired.

When your calorie intake is not meeting your body's needs, the protein you eat may end up being used for energy instead of all-important tissue repair. The body may even need to break down its own muscle to provide calories. If this happens, you become weak. To maintain strength and speed recovery, you must maintain an adequate intake of calories and protein. Generally, men require 2,700 calories per day and women need about 2,000. During illness, treatment, and recovery, both men and women should try to consume an additional 200 to 300 calories per day.

To maintain weight, a person must consume as many calories as the body uses each day. Many people with cancer find they are no longer as hungry as they used to be. They end up losing weight without really noticing. If you have lost a lot of weight already, your goal should be to maintain your weight for a while, and then start trying to gain. When you have been losing, just to maintain is going to be a struggle and will require some creative boosting of calories.

Hints to Boost Caloric Intake

- Add extra butter or margarine to foods. Just by melting two teaspoons of butter into potatoes or soup, you add an extra 90 calories. Serve bread hot so that more butter will melt into it.

- Nuts are high in calories and are a good source of protein.

- Mayonnaise has 100 calories per tablespoon. Use it in salads and on sandwiches. Extra mayonnaise on sandwiches adds moistness, which is often soothing to a sore mouth.

- Sour cream is also cool and moist as well as being loaded with calories (1 tablespoon = 70 calories). Try it on hot vegetables or added to gravies.

- Honey (1 tablespoon = 65 calories) can be spread on toast or used as a sweetener in coffee or cereal.

- High calorie snacks should be kept on hand: nuts, dried fruits, candy, popcorn,or crackers with cheese.

- Ice cream, at 145 calories per half cup, is a perfect high-calorie snack. When thrown in the blender with milk and fresh fruit, it makes a cool, soothing drink that is high in both protein and calories.

When You Don't Feel Like Eating

During treatment for cancer, sometimes you just don't feel like eating. Radiation and chemotherapy can interfere with proper appetite in many ways, including causing nausea and vomiting, feelings of fullness, mouth sores or sore throat, a bitter or metallic taste, and bowel problems.

On days when you just don't feel like eating, make sure your fluid intake remains high (6 to 8 glasses of fluid per day). This is especially important with most chemotherapy regimens.

When you do start feeling a little better, food still may not sound appealing. Many people with cancer have found that the following techniques make eating easier and more enjoyable:

Hints to Stimulate Appetite

Create the right atmosphere. If you are standing alone at the kitchen counter, it is easy to decide against eating, even though you know you should. Making meals a social affair stimulates the appetite. Set the table with placemats and flowers; play pleasant dinner music; and perhaps invite family and friends to join you. You will be more relaxed and may discover you are more hungry than you first thought.

Have a glass of wine or beer before a meal (with the doctor's approval). It is relaxing and can also be an appetite stimulant. Good odors may help. The smell of a fresh loaf of bread or cake baking in the oven can make you hungry for those foods.

Take advantage of the "up" times. When you're feeling good, eat well. This is also a good time to prepare meals that can be frozen and easily reheated on your down days. When you're feeling good, eat whenever you're hungry, even if it isn't at mealtime. All the nutrients you consume at these times will be stored for later use.

Make use of time savers. Some people don't have a problem with eating during chemotherapy, but they often feel too tired to cook. If this is the case, here are some suggestions:

- Let someone else do the cooking.
- Prepare a helper list of people who can shop, cook, set the

table, and clean up for you. Discuss the list with family members and post it where it can be seen by all.

- On high-energy days, cook large batches of food that can be frozen and used later. Add instructions so others can help you.

- Prepare and post a weekly menu including items that can be easily put together. Simple casseroles, hamburgers, frozen pizza, or TV dinners are all good, easy ideas.

- Accept gifts of food and offers of help from family and friends. If you can't use the food right away, freeze it.

- Use paper plates, napkins, and disposable silverware as often as necessary to save on dishwashing. Use disposable pans for cooking. (Foil containers from frozen dinners make excellent disposable pans).

Keep snacks on hand. Good ideas for easy snacks would be ice cream, peanut butter and crackers, pudding, peanuts, dried fruits, and canned milk shakes.

Concentrate on breakfast. The word breakfast actually means "break the fast." Although many people neglect this meal, most nutritionists consider it the most important meal of the day. Fortunately, morning is usually the time when people with cancer have the most energy and feel the most like eating. A good breakfast that includes all the four food groups (one egg, sausage, whole wheat toast, orange juice, and milk) is an excellent way to pack maximum nutrition into one meal.

Eat small, frequent meals. Instead of planning on three meals a day, eat just a little bit at a time, but eat more often. If weight loss has been a problem, be sure to ask yourself every two hours or so if you have eaten something lately. By eating nutritious snacks every few hours throughout the day, you can probably get your nutritional needs met without too much effort.

Treat yourself frequently to your favorite foods. Plan your weekly menus around foods that have always been your favorite. Many people mention chicken or spaghetti with meatballs as mainstays in their menu favorites.

At mealtime, eat solid foods before liquids. Liquids may fill you up before you have met your body's nutritional needs. Save the liquids for after the meal.

Exercise to stimulate yourj appetite. Try to take a short walk right before eating. Not only does it stimulate the appetite, but walking keeps your body in shape and reduces stress.

These last two suggestions are provided for family and friends of the person with cancer:

Don't talk about food constantly. Family members often become overly concerned about eating when they see the person with cancer losing weight. But this concern often feels like nagging to the patient who just isn't hungry. The family could "contract" one time of day when food is discussed. Outside of that one time, discussion of food should be off-limits. Comments like, "Oh, try a little of this," and "You're not eating enough," become irritating to someone who simply has no appetite.

Don't use the smorgasbord approach. Putting six or seven things in front of someone and then asking them to just have a little bit of something can actually turn the appetite off. Too much food is overwhelming. Since most people undergoing treatment can only eat a little bit at a time, it is better to offer a small portion of one item at frequent intervals throughout the day.

Side Effects From Cancer Treatment That Inhibit Good Nutrition

In addition to loss of appetite, people experience other side effects that interfere with the enjoyment of eating. The following hints may help relieve these symptoms.

Hints to Relieve Nausea and Vomiting

- Serve foods at room temperature.

- Take antinausea medicine one-half to one hour before eating.

- Eat small portions of low-fat foods such as applesauce or gelatin.

- Avoid nauseating food smells. Cold tuna salad is a good way to get high protein and avoid offensive food smells.

- Eat salty foods and avoid sweet foods.

- Eat dry foods (toast or crackers) in the morning.

- Drink clear, cool beverages (soda pop, juice, Kool-Aid).

- Rest after eating, but do not lie down flat for at least two hours.

- Avoid greasy, fried foods, both because of the smells and because they are hard on the stomach.

Hints to Relieve Mouth and Throat Problems

- Avoid eating highly acidic and spicy foods such as oranges or pizza.

- Try a softer diet. Many favorite foods can be put in a blender while they are still warm and come out tasting very good.

- Eat food lukewarm rather than hot or cold.

- Avoid alcohol and tobacco.

- Use a straw to make drinking easier.

- Soak foods in your beverage before eating. For example, soaking bread in milk makes it easier to chew and swallow.

- Avoid citrus fruit juices (grapefruit, pineapple, orange).

- Try the following foods, which are usually well tolerated: custards, Popsicles®, puddings, milk shakes, ice cream, eggnog, gelatin, and milk.

- Use butter, gravies, or sauces with food whenever possible.

- Suck on sugarless candy or ice chips.

Hints to Relieve a Bitter or Metallic Taste

- If meat doesn't taste right, substitute chicken, turkey, eggs, or dairy products.

- Eat foods that leave their own tastes in your mouth such as fresh fruits or hard candies.

- Drink more liquids.

- Eat foods cold or at room temperature. They'll taste better.

- To add flavor to meats, marinate them in sweet fruit juices, sweet wines, or Italian dressing.

- If you are not having problems with a sore mouth or throat, try strongly flavored foods (pizza or tacos).

Hints to Relieve Diarrhea

- Avoid foods with high-fiber content, such as fresh fruits or vegetables or whole-grain cereals and breads.

- Consume fluids between meals, not during meals.

- Eat small, frequent meals.

- Serve foods warm or at room temperature.

- Avoid gas-forming foods such as beer, beans, cabbage, broccoli, cauliflower, gum, coffee, and too many sweets.

- Try applesauce, cheese, cottage cheese, gelatin, toast, tea.

Hints to Relieve Constipation

- Include a variety of fiber-rich foods in your diet: fruits, vegetables, whole grains, nuts, and popcorn.

- Add one or two tablespoons of bran to foods.

- Include prunes and prune juice in your daily diet.

- Drink plenty of liquids. Hot liquids stimulate bowel activity.

- Take a laxative or stool softener if prescribed by your doctor.

- If possible, try to exercise a little each day.

Nutritional Supplements

Despite all their best efforts, some people are still unable to get enough protein and calories into their daily diet. Because adequate nutrition is essential during treatment, most health care providers recommend a commercial nutritional supplement to those people. Many different brands of supplements are available, at either a pharmacy or grocery store. Those interested should ask their doctor or nurse to make a recommendation. In some cases, if the doctor writes a prescription for supplements, insurance will cover the cost.

Managing Other Side Effects

Cancer and its various treatments can cause other side effects in addition to those related to diet and appetite. Again, remember that individual reactions vary. No two people respond to radiation or chemotherapy in quite the same way. Some people experience very few or no side effects. Others have serious problems. Following are some of the most commonly reported side effects of cancer and its treatment.

Nausea and Vomiting

The most exciting news about this side effect is that it is occurring far less frequently these days. Why? A new medication called ondansetron (marketed under the name Zofran®) relieves most instances of queasy stomach. The drug works by intercepting the connection of the neurotransmitter serotonin to receptors in the gastrointestinal tract and brain. This interception breaks the nerve impulse that triggers vomiting.

And there's more good news. Unlike traditional antinausea medications, which sometimes produce drowsiness or agitation, ondansetron appears to have no major side effects. Researchers continue to work on the best way to administer the drug.

Even after 10 years, Bill hadn't forgotten his stay in the intensive care unit after his first chemotherapy, and the subsequent four months of treatment. The memories weren't all pleasant. He wasn't looking forward to four more months of the same thing. This time, he was pleasantly surprised. "That Zofran is a miracle drug," Bill says. "After sitting in the outpatient clinic all day getting the drugs, I could drive home, jump on my lawn tractor, and go to work. I was never nauseated, and usually not even tired." And Bill was receiving some powerful drugs, combinations that in the past almost always caused nausea and vomiting. Zofran made the difference.

Two additional benefits surface from this new drug. First, chemotherapy success depends on patient cooperation. Several studies have shown that nausea and vomiting often cause a patient to refuse further treatment. When nausea and vomiting do not occur, patients are more likely to continue on a high-dose drug regimen because they feel better and stronger and their nutritional needs aren't being interrupted.

Another benefit is that of alleviating anxiety and fear surrounding chemotherapy. Bill's wife, Laura, is a good example. "If I ever got cancer, I wouldn't be afraid to go in and have chemotherapy now," she says. "I could never have said that before. And if I hadn't actually been living with Bill and seen how he reacted, I'm not sure I would believe it yet."

Many people still don't believe it. For instance, even though only 20 percent of women receiving the most widely prescribed chemo combinations for breast cancer—cyclophosphamide, methotrexate, and fluorouracil—report nausea and vomiting, anxiety over chemotherapy continues. Researchers studying anticipatory nausea and vomiting (having symptoms before receiving chemotherapy) find that the attitude and behavior of patients in clinical trials doesn't equate with the success of the antinausea drug they are given. Many people still tend to display a high level of anxiety regarding chemotherapy, as exhibited by these anticipatory symptoms.

Research continues in an attempt to find new ways to manage anticipatory nausea without the use of drugs. For some people, strenuous exercise just before treatment has a calming effect. For those who are adept at relaxation and visualization, using such techniques before and during treatment sometimes reduces anticipatory symptoms.

Finally, could these anticipatory symptoms be caused by something more complex than just a reaction to the medical treatment program? Researchers are now studying patients' mental health, family dynamics, and other psychological factors in an attempt to answer that question. People from families that are emotionally well tend to weather cancer treatment better than people from dysfunctional families. Researchers would like to know why so they can develop ways to bolster the emotional wellness of the patients from dysfunctional environments.

Hair Loss

Radiation and chemotherapy are both very effective in killing cancer cells. Unfortunately, they also can damage normal cells in the process. The normal cells that are most susceptible to damage are those that multiply rapidly, such as hair follicles. For many people, the anxiety about chemotherapy relates to hair loss, not nausea and vomiting. No one can predict exactly how the hair will be affected, but a doctor, nurse, or pharmacist can offer some ideas on what to expect based on the type of drug and the amount the patient receives.

Hair loss usually begins within a few days or weeks of treatment. Most people first notice the hair loss when they are combing, brushing, or washing their hair. Sometimes huge chunks of hair fall to the shower floor. Other times, the hair comes out gradually while brushing. The hair breaks off at or near the skin, and the skull may become tender. If hair continues to grow, it often is dull and dry.

By the third cycle of chemotherapy, people usually know whether or not their hair is going to be affected. Some lose just a little hair. Others become totally bald. And some may keep the hair on their heads but lose body hair. The good news is that hair loss resulting from chemotherapy is almost always reversible. Sometimes new hair begins to grow back even while the person is still being treated. When the hair does grow back, it is often thick and soft, frequently wavy or curly. Some say their hair is more beautiful the second time around.

During the period of hair loss and baldness, people sometimes feel self-conscious and depressed. Many consider hair loss the most upsetting side effect of treatment. Hair is an important part of a person's self-concept. Barbara Walters once said, "If my hair looks good, the rest of my day will go well." For many women, having a "bad hair day" is depressing; having no hair at all for months is traumatic. After having your self-esteem fractured by a cancer diagnosis, hair loss can only serve to magnify the loss. But, difficult as it may seem at first, people do manage to adjust.

Dave chose to use an ice pack-type cap on his head while undergoing chemotherapy. He was warned it might not have any effect, but he was fortunate and ended up with only partial hair loss. He wore the cap through the treatment and for 30 minutes afterward.

Malinda was not so lucky. Her hair fell out two weeks after her second chemotherapy treatment. Her friends rallied round to help her adjust by taking her shopping for the right wig. "My hairdresser even took my wigs home and worked on them to make them look more like me. Then we went scarf shopping together." Malinda began experimenting with ways to wrap her head in scarves. When she went to a party wearing a unique, colorful scarf and large loop earrings, one person commented, "That woman has such an interesting look. What country is she from?" Malinda managed to retain her flare for fashion. For her, it was important to look good even when she was feeling bad.

To match hair color and style, buying a wig before starting chemotherapy is a good idea. Wigs are a tax-deductible medical expense and may also be covered by some health insurance policies. Usually a good synthetic wig is preferable to real hair because it is less expensive to buy and maintain, it washes and dries better, and it is cooler to wear. Although hair loss can be depressing and no wig is an adequate substitute for real hair, it is important to remember that the wig will be necessary for only a short time.

When Malinda's hair started growing back, she gave up the wig almost immediately. "My attitude was to bloom where you are planted. Make the best of what you have." Fortunately, "punk" hairdos were popular at the time, so the half inch of auburn fuzz all over Malinda's head was right in style. "It was actually kind of fun. I never would have dared go out with a hairdo like that before all this happened."

Malinda made the best of a bad situation and soon had a full head of hair again. But when there is radiation to the brain, most doctors and nurses are pessimistic about the possibility of the hair growing back. Hair loss from radiation to the head usually occurs in patches that coincide with the areas or the most intense radiation. This differs from hair loss from chemotherapy, which tends to be of a more general nature.

Debbie's thick, blond hair began falling out during her radiation therapy. Because the radiation was mainly to the upper side of her head, that was where most of the hair loss occurred. By the time treatment was complete, Debbie had several bald spots. Hair loss was particularly devastating for Debbie, since she worked in cosmetics and took great pride in her looks. In the beginning, she was totally turned off by wigs and refused to look at them. She compensated by wearing wide headbands that were color coordinated with her clothing. But as time went on, she became more and more depressed about her looks.

Finally, she gave in and bought a wig. The first day she wore it, her mood brightened. "For the first time in a long time, I actually looked forward to going out of the house. Guys started looking at me again." Debbie realized her wig was no substitute for her own hair, but it made her look normal, and that made her feel normal.

In time, Debbie defied the odds and got almost all of her hair back. When it had grown out to about one-half inch, she had her hairdresser cut all of her hair to that length, leaving a few long tendrils of hair at the nape of her neck. "The people at work didn't even blink an eye at that haircut. When you're selling cosmetics, people expect you to look a little different." The only drawback to Debbie's new hair was its color. "For the first time in my life, I was a dishwater blonde, and I hated it." For some people, the new hair comes in darker. For others, it may come in lighter. Straight hair becomes curly. No one can predict ahead of time exactly what color or texture someone's new hair will be.

After radiation treatments, Dick didn't get much new hair at all. But being in remission from lung cancer for more than 15 years compensates for the loss.

Blood Counts

Three different types of blood cells are produced in the bone marrow: white blood cells, red blood cells, and platelets. Because blood cells are among the most rapidly dividing cells, they are particularly sensitive to the effects of anticancer drugs. Therefore, doctors take frequent blood samples to monitor the effect of the drugs on the bone marrow. It is important to be aware of the symptoms that may signal a bone marrow problem. Those symptoms are outlined in the following paragraphs, along with more information on blood cell types.

White Blood Cells (WBC)

White blood cells help protect the body by fighting infection-causing bacteria. The cells that immediately rush to the site of any infection are called neutrophils. Normally, the bone marrow responds by speeding up production of neutrophils to replace those used to fight the infection.

Chemotherapy that destroys immune cells is particularly devastating to neutrophils. The colony-stimulating factor (CSF) rG-CSF stimulates the production of neutrophils that fight bacteria. This CSF is used most often in patients receiving myelosuppressive therapy. For bone marrow transplant patients, rGM-CSF is used, which also stimulates production of cells that fight bacteria and fungi, and cells involved in the body's allergic response.

Not all people will receive CSFs, but anyone receiving chemotherapy should be particularly cautious. Watch for fevers (temperature over 100 ° F), colds, rashes, cuts that get infected, or any itching or burning in the genital area. During times when the white blood cell count is low, some steps can be taken to reduce the chance of infection.

Precautions When WBC Is Low

- Wash your hands often throughout the day.

- Avoid crowds and people with colds, coughs, and other infectious diseases.

- Do no tear or cut your nail cuticles.

- To avoid breaks in the skin, use an electric razor.

- Take a warm shower every day and pat your skin dry.

- If you cut or scrape your skin, wash immediately with warm soap and water.

- Avoid raw vegetables and fruit that can't be peeled.

- Avoid flowers and plants; they are sources of bacteria and fungi.

- Don't garden; don't clean cat litter boxes or bird cages.

- Avoid undercooked meat and poultry.

Even with the best precautions, infections can still occur. Be on the lookout for the following signs of infection, and report them immediately to your doctor:

Signs of Infection

- Fever over 100° F.

- Chills.

- Sweating, especially at night.

- Loose bowels.

- Burning sensation when urinating.

- Severe cough or sore throat.

Red Blood Cells (RBC)

Red blood cells carry oxygen to all parts of the body. A decreased red blood cell count can result in anemia, caused by body tissues not getting enough oxygen to do their work. If your red blood cell count gets too low, your doctor may advise having a blood transfusion or may prescribe a colony-stimulating factor called r-HuEPO, which will stimulate the production of red blood cells. Symptoms of anemia include shortness of breath, weakness, and fatigue. You can do several things to help alleviate these symptoms.

Precautions When RBC Is Low

- Get plenty of rest, and plan your day to conserve energy.

- Add more green, leafy vegetables, liver, and red meat to your diet.

- Move slowly to avoid dizziness.

Platelets

Platelets help blood to clot, and they stop bleeding when the skin has been cut. If the platelet count is low, a person may bleed or bruise more easily or a rash of small blood blisters can develop under the skin. Some people develop internal bleeding. To avoid problems when the platelet count is low, consider the following suggestions:

Precautions When Platelets Are Low

- Do not take any medication without a doctor's approval.

- Do not drink alcohol without a doctor's approval.

- Use cotton swabs instead of a toothbrush to clean your teeth and mouth.

- Be extra careful when using knives or tools.

- Be careful not to burn yourself when ironing or cooking.

- Avoid contact sports that might result in injury.

Report any unusual bleeding or bruising to your doctor. If your platelet count gets too low, a transfusion of platelets may be necessary. Research is being done to identify a colony-stimulating factor that will stimulate production of platelets.

Monitoring Blood Counts During Bone Marrow Transplants

Most of Dave's five weeks in the hospital revolved around constant monitoring of his red and white blood cell counts (including the neutrophils) and his platelets. During the first six days, he received high-dose chemotherapy, then he had two days of rest before the actual bone marrow transplant. Although the concept of transplant conjures up thoughts of donor organs arriving in airplanes and large teams of doctors in white coats, the bone marrow transplant is actually a relatively simple procedure.

Dave's marrow had been frozen up until the morning of his transplant, so the oncologist thawed the bags of frozen marrow in a hot-water bath. When the marrow reached body temperature, the doctor drew the marrow up into 60-cc. syringes and brought them into the room. Then it was just a matter of connecting the syringe to the tubing of Dave's catheter and emptying the marrow back into his bloodstream. Within minutes, the marrow would act like miniature homing pigeons and magically circulate through Dave's system, eventually finding its way back to the marrow cavity where it was originally harvested.

In his journal, Dave noted: "The injection of the bone marrow through my catheter seemed to be a very straightforward and solemn process. Even though the hospital staff had downplayed the transplant procedure, I was aware of how seriously they were handling the task at hand." Dave's entire family was with him, and after the procedure, they played Bob Seger's *Katmandu* on the CD player and everyone danced. Dave even managed to wiggle his toes to the beat of the music.

The next day his white blood count dropped to 500, and within two days it was below 200. Doctors were concerned about a sore that wasn't healing and experimented with different antibiotics. Within four days, Dave had his first platelet transfusion, an uneventful procedure, except that it made him very sleepy. His second platelet transfusion gave him a severe case of the chills. His nurse immediately responded with Demerol, but Dave was still shaking, both physically and emotionally. In his journal, he noted, "I don't know how long I was shaking, but it seemed like it wasn't ever going to stop. And I have to say that I had an emotional reaction, too. It was *deja vu*—those memories of my prediagnosis experience came flooding back." The next time he was scheduled to receive platelets, he asked the nurse to wait until his wife and daughter were with him.

Typically, bone marrow transplant patients require platelet transfusions for about four weeks after the transplant. By now, Dave was also receiving red blood cell transfusions as well. But he had to rely on his own system to supply the white blood cells, since his transplant took place before doctors were routinely using colony-stimulating factors to promote production of white blood cells. Dave's white cell counts stayed down between 100 and 200 for quite some time, and by his seventeenth day of hospitalization, he had developed a fever of 101.5° F. But his medical team kept it under control, and by the twentieth day, he seemed to be rallying.

"This may be the start of my bone marrow turnaround," Dave noted in his journal. "I got dressed today, complete with golf cap to top my thinning pate and windbreaker to stave off the chill. My line for the day is, 'Get that IV team over here to unhook me and I'm gone.'"

Although Dave felt well enough to go home that day, he was in the hospital another 16 days so his white blood counts and particularly his neutrophils could be constantly monitored. Each day his journal documented the vacillating numbers, and each day his hopes spiked or fell along with those numbers. Finally, by day 29, he resigned himself to "waiting patiently for the bone marrow to do its job and not making unrealistic plans to get out of here." Seven days later, Dave was released, just in time for Thanksgiving.

Pain

Albert Schweitzer said, "Pain is a more terrible lord of mankind than even death himself." When people first learn they have cancer, a common reaction is, "But how will I deal with the pain?" People believe pain will always be a part of cancer. This is rarely true in cancer's early stages, and it is not necessarily true in advanced cancer.

Pain occurs when your body sends a message to your nervous system saying, "Something is wrong." Damaged tissue sets off the alarm, which runs like an electrical impulse through the spinal cord to the thalamus, the sensory center of the brain. Next, it moves on to the cortex, the brain's outer layer. Now the person feels the location and intensity of the pain, and the brain responds by sending signals back down the spinal cord, releasing chemicals like endorphins to diminish the pain.

Cancer pain depends on the type of cancer, the stage of the disease, and the individual's pain threshold. There are several different causes of pain:

- Pressure exerted on a nerve by tumor.
- Infection or inflammation.
- An organ, tube, or blood vessel that is blocked.
- Pressure caused by cancer cells that have spread to the bone.

- Side effects from chemotherapy or radiation.

- Emotional responses to the disease, such as tension or anxiety.

Pain is relieved when pain signals are blocked as they travel from the site of the injury to the brain. When pain does occur, it can almost always be managed with drugs or a combination of drug and nondrug therapies. But for pain to be managed most effectively, the person with cancer must be able to accurately describe it. Many people are afraid to speak up and admit that their pain is intense. The health care team has no way of knowing how severe the pain is until they are told. So don't hesitate to tell doctors and nurses exactly how you feel. You have every right to ask for pain relief, and today most people who have pain, even severe pain, can be relieved.

Although pain is sometimes difficult to explain, precisely descriptive words make it easier for the medical professional to determine the cause. For instance, if someone describes a pain as being "intermittent, burning, and throbbing," this is often a clue that a nerve is involved.

The following chart lists includes some things your doctor or nurse needs to know about your pain:

Pain Inventory

- Where do you feel the pain?

- When did the pain begin?

- What does it feel like? Is it sharp? Dull? Throbbing? Steady?

- Does it stay in one place or move around?

- What relieves your pain?

- What makes your pain worse?

- What have you tried for pain relief?

- Did it work?

- Is the pain constant? If not, how often does it occur?

- How long does the pain last? Is it constant? Intermittent?

- How intense is it? Use the line below to describe.

No pain   Worst pain you can
                                                    imagine

1   2   3   4   5   6   7   8   9   10

Sometimes it is helpful to keep a diary that you can refer to the next time you see your doctor. Be sure to include any activity that seems to increase or decrease the pain, how frequently you take pain medication, the name and amount of the medication, and whether you take medication before the pain starts or only when you are in pain. Be sure to assign a number from the pain-intensity rating scale that best describes your pain.

Eliminating Pain with Medication

Pain medicine falls into three major categories: nonnarcotics (aspirin, Tylenol®); anti-inflammatory drugs (ibuprofin, Motrin®); and narcotics (codeine, Demerol®, morphine). When pain is mild to moderate, the nonnarcotics and anti-inflammatory drugs are often effective. However, people on chemotherapy should avoid aspirin and should always check with the doctor before taking any over-the-counter medication.

Often the medication prescribed by your doctor does not do the job. Why is this? Poor pain control is sometimes the result of poor medical education. Doctors are taught how to treat cancer, but not the pain of cancer. Some doctors and nurses may under-utilize medications because they fear the patient's becoming addicted. Finally, pain medications may be inadequate because the person in pain doesn't speak up and clearly describe the pain.

The following are some points to remember about using medication to control pain:

The medication must be equal to the pain. There are three types of pain: mild, moderate, and severe. And there are three classifications of drugs for mild, moderate, and severe pain. Taking a drug designed for mild pain when you are experiencing severe pain is like using a squirt gun on a house fire. No amount of medication will be able to touch the pain. Be honest and specific about the degree of pain. Otherwise, the prescribed drug may be inappropriate.

Medication must be taken before the pain becomes intense. Many people tend to "tough it out," and wait until the pain gets really bad before taking medication. Once the pain has traveled from the original site through all the nerve receptors in the body and into the brain, it takes a long time for medication to reverse that cycle. For most people, it is best to take medication on a regular schedule (every three or four hours), around the clock to prevent the pain cycle from starting.

Pain medications come in many forms. Most often they are given orally as pills or in liquid form, intravenously, through a skin patch, or by a rectal suppository. Some pills now provide pain relief for up to 12 hours, and a patch can be effective for as long as three days.

Ambulatory pumps give patients more control over pain. Patient - controlled analgesia (PCA) machines, or ambulatory pumps, permit patients to administer their own doses of medication (up to a safe maximum limit) as needed. The PCA can also be adjusted so the medication is automatically dispensed according to a predetermined dosage. One study found that patients who administer their own medication report less pain, use pain medication over a shorter time period, and require less drugs in total than those who receive their medication from a health professional.

Narcotic pain relievers may have side effects. People may experience drowsiness, nausea, and vomiting when taking narcotics. Other drugs can be combined with the pain medications to decrease these side effects as well as enhance the potency of the narcotic.

Morphine is no longer considered a "last effort" drug. The American College of Physicians, the American Medical Association, and the World Health Organization all agree that oral morphine is the drug of choice for chronic, severe pain. It is a myth that morphine use leads to addiction. People with severe cancer pain are not using morphine for kicks. They need it. The chemical make-up of oral morphine closely resembles the body's own pain-killing endorphins. When pain becomes less severe, the person's need for the drug automatically decreases.

When pain is so severe that the quality of life is severely impaired, more extreme measures may be necessary. Sometimes a neurosurgeon or anesthesiologist will perform an epidural block, in which a small tube is placed in tissue around the spinal cord and medication is delivered directly to the nerve causing the pain. The medication may be morphine, or a similar narcotic, a local anesthetic, or a steroid. In other cases, neurosurgery creates a nerve block or completely destroys the nerves that transmit pain, giving patients total and permanent relief.

In most cases, the right drug in the right dose given at the right time and in the right way relieves 85 to 90 percent of pain. People who are knowledgeable about their pain and assertive enough to ask for what they need usually achieve an acceptable level of pain control over long periods of time.

Eliminating Pain with Nondrug Therapies

Football players do it. Olympic athletes do it. Women in childbirth do it. They all use some form of nondrug therapy to relieve pain. While drugs are the primary source of pain relief for many cancer patients, the following nondrug therapies also help patients better manage their pain.

Education. Research has shown that when patients know approximately when pain will end, they can tolerate it better. Patients should find out in advance what type of pain is normal, the cause of the pain, how long it is likely to last, and what will be done to relieve it.

Distraction. The injured football player is probably the best example of the power of distraction. He is so distracted by the continuing activity of the game, he doesn't have time to notice the pain signals his brain is sending. Cancer patients can watch movies, listen to soothing music, talk to friends, work on a hobby, or engage in some physical activity as ways to distract their thoughts from pain.

Relaxation and Imagery. Once only scoffed at as primitive religious rituals, activities that heighten mind control have been widely studied and have proven to be very successful pain-control techniques for some people. Relaxation involves a series of muscle tensing and relaxing exercises or breathing exercises designed to induce a sense of calm. When combined with imagery (taking a trip in your mind to a pleasant, safe, relaxing environment), relaxation can effectively calm patients and help them control their pain.

Biofeedback. By helping people recognize, modify, and control certain involuntary habits or bodily responses, biofeedback can ease anxiety, tension, and muscle pain.

Hypnosis. A skilled therapist can use distraction and imagery to put a patient in a passive, trancelike state that ignores involuntary body responses and blocks pain. Hypnosis works especially well in combination with medication.

Physical stimulation. This technique uses pressure (usually some form of massage), heat, cold, vibration, electrical stimulation, or menthol preparations. The philosophy is to provide a different, competing physical sensation that will block the sensation of pain.

Pain is not inevitable, and it is almost always controllable. Be patient and work closely with your health care professionals. It may take time to identify the exact cause and work out the proper combination of drug and nondrug therapies to relieve your pain.

Weakness and Fatigue

During cancer treatment, the body's cells are constantly in an evolutionary state. This constant regeneration can cause fatigue. In addition, low blood counts can also be the culprit on days when people are feeling particularly tired.

Both Debbie and Lothair complained of being totally wiped out while undergoing radiation therapy. Lothair napped every afternoon and spent much of his time in quiet activity, either reading or listening to classical music. When Debbie became aware of how exhausted she was getting during treatment, she arranged to work only part time.

The body uses a great deal of energy during radiation therapy. And it takes additional energy to make the daily trips to the hospital or clinic. Most people receive radiation five days a week for several weeks. This rigorous treatment schedule and the effects of treatment itself tend to make people very tired. These suggestions may make dealing with fatigue easier:

- Ask less of yourself. Rest in your leisure time.
- Nap during the day, and get more sleep at night.

137

- If you are still working full time, schedule treatment for the end of the day.

- If possible, take a few weeks off during treatment or work reduced hours.

- Ask for help. Friends and relatives want to be helpful, and this is the perfect opportunity. They can help with shopping, housework, and child care. Also, ask someone to drive you to treatment to help conserve your energy.

Skin Problems

Skin problems can result from either chemotherapy or radiation. Chemotherapy can cause redness, itching, peeling, dryness, and acne. After radiation, skin in the area being radiated may become dry and itchy. Today, this occurs less frequently because newer equipment allows for deeper rays and smaller, more frequent doses. Sometimes the skin darkens or looks sunburned after radiation. The therapy team watches closely for symptoms that could signal the need for a change in treatment.

People with skin problems might benefit from the following suggestions:

- For acne, keep your face clean and dry, and use over-the-counter medicated creams or soaps.

- For dry skin, apply light baby oil.

- For itching or excess moisture, dust your skin with corn starch.

- Do not rub, scrub, or scratch sensitive spots.

- Do not use home remedies such as powders, creams, or salves during radiation treatment and for several weeks after.

- Ask your doctor to suggest an acceptable lotion to use.

- Tell your doctor about any blisters, skin cracks, or excess moisture you notice during radiation.

- Inform your doctor or nurse of any sudden or severe rash, hives, or itching you have after chemotherapy.

Skin problems can be particularly difficult for women, and specific kinds of makeup and lotions are sometimes advised. In addition, many women start to question their attractiveness about this time. Personal appearance affects self-image and psychological well-being, and when people with cancer look in the mirror, sometimes they don't see what they used to see. The face in the mirror reflects not only skin problems, but also fatigue, hair loss, weight gain, or weight loss.

To help women deal with some of these problems, the Look Good...Feel Better© program was developed by the Cosmetic, Toiletry, and Fragrance Association (CTFA) Foundation in partnership with the American Cancer Society (ACS) and the National Cosmetology Association (NCA). Together, they offer:

- Education by volunteer cosmetologists and beauty advisers

- Complimentary makeup kits for every participant

- Free program materials (videos and pamphlets)

Volunteer cosmetologists evaluate skin and hair needs and teach beauty techniques to counteract appearance-related side effects of cancer treatment. To learn more about Look Good... Feel Better©, contact your local American Cancer Society office or call 1-800-395-LOOK.

Dental Problems

A strict program of oral health care is vital during chemotherapy and radiation. Chemotherapy affects the rapidly growing cells of the lining of the mouth, and the tissues become more susceptible to infection. Radiation treatments to the brain, mouth, neck, or upper chest also affect the teeth, gums, and other mouth tissues. A few simple precautions will help prevent or control mouth problems:

- Before starting your treatment, see your dentist for a complete checkup.

- Tell the dentist about your impending therapy. A consultation may be in order between the dentist and your therapist regarding proper dental care. Because radiation treatments increase the chances of getting cavities, you may need to see your dentist often during treatment.

- Clean your teeth and gums thoroughly but gently with a soft brush after meals and at least once more daily. Brushing too hard can damage soft tissues.

- Do not use commercial mouthwash; the alcohol content has a drying effect on mouth tissues.

- Use a fluoride toothpaste that contains no abrasives; apply fluoride to your teeth daily.

- Make a soothing, effective mouth rinse with 1 teaspoon of baking soda in 1 cup of warm water.

Urinary Tract Problems

Some anticancer drugs may cause the urine to change color. Don't be alarmed if your urine is red while you're taking doxorubicin (Adriamycin) or daunorubicin, or bright yellow if you take methotrexate. The urine also can take on a strong, medicine-like odor from certain drugs.

Continue drinking plenty of fluids to ensure good urine flow and prevent problems. Eight glasses of water a day is advisable. Ask your doctor if the drugs you are taking are among those that can damage the kidney or bladder.

Sexual Problems

Any discussion of side effects should include sexual changes that occur either from cancer and its treatment or from medications. Many drugs used in chemotherapy cause changes in the reproductive system. This can mean sterility in men or possible temporary loss of menstrual periods or infertility in women. Because reactions to the chemicals vary, young women should thoroughly discuss contraception with their doctor to prevent an unwanted pregnancy while undergoing chemotherapy. Young men may want to consider sperm banking before treatment if they think they may be interested in starting a family later.

Whether it is the cancer itself, the surgery, the treatment, or general anxiety, many people experience decreased libido during this time. Chapter 6, Exploring Self-Esteem and Intimacy, covers the topic of sexual problems comprehensively and offers suggestions to help people remain intimate even though their sexual needs have changed.

Residual Side Effects of Cancer Treatments

For many people, infertility and sterility from chemotherapy are irreversible. Dick suffered permanent hair loss from radiation. Both Bill and Dave still have some numbness in their fingers and toes.

Bone marrow transplant patients must be particularly watchful for infection. Fungal and viral infections are not uncommon, are difficult to treat, and can cause pneumonia. The chemotherapy administered during the transplant destroys T-cells and depletes antibodies responsible for keeping viruses in check. Viral infections are most common during the first 12 months after a transplant, but they may occur as late as two or more years after transplant.

Dave was surprised to learn that 20 to 40 percent of bone marrow transplant patients come down with the Varicella Zoster virus (VZV), better known as shingles, and he was unfortunate enough to be one of them. This is the same virus that causes chicken pox, and high-dose chemotherapy significantly reduces a patient's existing immunity to this virus. Shingles is an itching, blistering skin rash extending along any one of the body's nerve branches. The virus can be quite painful, but early treatment can reduce the pain.

Know What to Expect–It Helps

Daily health care takes on a whole new dimension for the person with cancer. But dealing with the added health care problems is far easier when there are no surprises waiting around the corner. People tend to cope better when they understand some of the health problems that may or may not occur during the course of their disease and treatment.

If you have no side effects, consider yourself lucky. Sometimes the drugs are able to do their work without causing discomfort. Remember that the severity of the side effects has nothing to do with the effectiveness of the treatment. You can have a very successful treatment program and still feel good.

Suggested Reading

To learn more about topics discussed in Chapter 3, the following reading material is recommended:

Aker, Saundra N., and Polly Lenssen. *A Guide to Good Nutrition During and After Chemotherapy and Radiation.* Clinical Nutrition Program, E211, Fred Hutchinson Cancer Research Center, 1124 Columbia, Seattle, WA. 98104, 1988.

Bruning, Nancy. *Coping With Chemotherapy: How to Take Care of Yourself While Chemotherapy Takes Care of the Cancer.* New York: Ballantine Books, 1993. A comprehensive compilation of all aspects of chemotherapy told in a helpful, personal way by a cancer survivor.

Dodd, Marylin. *Managing the Side Effects of Chemotherapy and Radiation.* New York: Prentice Hall, 1987.

Fishman, Joan, R.D., M.S., and Barbara Anrod. *Something's Got to Taste Good: The Cancer Patient's Cookbook.* New York: Andrews and McNeel, Inc.; Paperback, Signet, 1982. Recipes that are easy to prepare, yet high in protein and calories.

Kalter, Suzy. *Looking Up: The Complete Guide to Looking Good and Feeling Good for the Recovering Cancer Patient.* New York: McGraw-Hill, 1987.

Noyes, Diane Doan, and Peggy Mellody. *Beauty and Cancer.* A.C. Press, 1988.

Ramstack, Janet L., and Ernest H. Rosenbaum. *Nutrition for the Chemotherapy Patient.* Palo Alto: Bull Publishing, 1990.

Wilson, J.R. *Non-Chew Cookbook.* Glenwood Springs, CO: Wilson Publishing Company, Inc. (P.O. Box 2190), 1985.

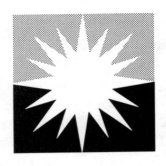

"If you use too much of your

energy in resisting

the stresses of life,

it's like running your car

and keeping the brakes on

at the same time.

You'll wear it out more rapidly."

Hans Selye
Stress Without Distress

CHAPTER FOUR

KEEPING ACTIVE IN MIND AND BODY

Bill started by unhooking his IV bottle from the stand and carrying it while he ran up two flights of stairs. Against the advice of the nursing staff, he was doing push-ups less than two weeks after surgery. "Another lesson my dad always preached was that motion is sacred," Bill says. "If you lie around too long and then get up, you won't be able to walk outside and back without getting all tired out."

Malinda asked her mother to massage her arm and shoulder even before the sedation from her surgery had worn off. As soon as she was able, she started range-of-motion exercises with her arm to get the muscles back in shape, then joined the local YWCA Encore swimming and discussion group for women with breast cancer.

For Dick, regaining the use of his working arm was all important. "The doctor couldn't believe it the day he walked in and saw me with that arm up over my head. They started calling me the miracle cure. But I had just decided to get my arm healthy. And I did."

The Circle of Wellness

Cancer and its treatment presented all ten people in this book with a variety of challenges. Bill, Malinda, and Dick didn't waste any time trying to compensate for and get beyond those challenges. They all seemed to define wellness in a broad sense, recognizing that it is much more than simply being free of cancer. Can you have cancer and still be healthy? The I CAN COPE philosophy is that cancer and healthy are not mutually exclusive and wellness is not measured on the physical scale alone. Wellness includes not only physical health, but emotional, intellectual, social, and spiritual health as well.

Emotional Wellness

Bill came from a close-knit family. He had always been encouraged to share feelings openly. He was with his parents when he learned about his cancer, and they have emotionally supported him 100 percent from the moment of diagnosis until the present. His father worked with Bill to find the right doctors. His mother, a nurse, helped him understand chemotherapy and what to expect. They brought him to their farm and nurtured him through a difficult recovery after his first week in the hospital for treatment. Such unconditional, loving support fosters emotional wellness. He entered the cancer experience with a healthy self-esteem and knew he could count on his family for stability and direction during the stressful times. Throughout his ordeal, his upbringing and basic personality helped him maintain a healthy, yet realistic, sense of optimism.

Dave's wife and daughters also contributed to his emotional wellness. His older daughter, who had been living on the East Coast, returned to live in Minnesota while Dave went through treatment and hospitalization for bone marrow transplant. When he entered the hospital, she gave him a journal with the inscription: "This journal is so you can document your journey toward the cure." During his six-week hospitalization, Dave filled the journal with notations about backgammon and cribbage games with his daughters and shared meals with his wife. They spent many evenings laughing together over humorous videos supplied by the girls or by family friends. On the day he received his bone marrow back, his older daughter wrote the following poem:

Your bone marrow is back, and here to stay;
It was definitely a family day.
Aunty, Mom, Krista, and Kira rooted and shouted hooray;
Now if only the sardine smell would go away!

Clearly, this kind of emotional support helped fuel Dave's already healthy optimism and carried him through his long hospital ordeal.

Unlike Bill and Dave, Debbie and Malinda had to fight for emotional wellness. Debbie remembered her years at home as tumultuous, marked by lack of communication and discord. She blamed no one; that's just the way it was. She left home at a young age and seldom returned. When cancer entered her life, her family seemed uncomfortable discussing it. They didn't have a history of expressing feelings. Debbie felt a new loneliness.

Malinda, married only four years before her cancer was discovered, struggled to pretend she was well for her husband's benefit. He seemed to feel cheated that his young wife had cancer, and initially this made her feel guilty. When they were separated, she went so far as to carefully time her trip to Louisiana so she would be visiting him at a time when she wouldn't be wearing the portable chemotherapy pump. But despite her courageous attempt to hide her illness, the seriousness of her condition soon became apparent. Her husband didn't seem emotionally capable of being the support she needed.

Intellectual and Social Wellness

Attending I CAN COPE classes promoted the intellectual and social wellness of all these individuals. Knowledge is power: the more you know, the less you fear. John knew what to expect from his colon cancer because he had already attended the classes after Hazel's breast cancer was discovered. Debbie was ignorant about all aspects of cancer until she attended I CAN COPE. And for Debbie, the accepting social environment created by class participants and facilitators afforded her an opportunity to establish new kinds of intimate relationships. When she and Malinda met at I CAN COPE, what began as a simple social interaction developed into a strong bond that ended up giving both women great emotional strength.

Intellectual wellness confirms that the mind is still healthy and can continue to learn despite physical illness. Social wellness is characterized by the recognition that friendships, social activities, and other affiliations keep a person involved in life instead of alienated from it.

Spiritual Wellness

No matter what your belief system is, cancer undeniably creates a spiritual crisis in a person's life. This confrontation with mortality nudges people into a journey of self-discovery, which often starts with the question: "What does it all mean, and what is my purpose here?" For some the journey is easier than others.

Debbie was pragmatic about her diagnosis from the start. She always believed it happened for a reason and was constantly searching for ways to assign meaning to the experience. She considered a career change, perhaps going back to school and finding a way to help others. She volunteered at a crisis phone center. Although she was raised Catholic, she had fallen away from her roots and dabbled in nontraditional religions. Yet during a later hospitalization, Debbie accepted Holy Communion. She was searching for spiritual wellness.

Like Debbie, most people with cancer are striving to make meaning out of chaos. In Victor Frankl's book, *Man's Search for Meaning*, he postulates that people who find meaning in their lives tend to be stronger survivors. Successful survivors often discover inner resources that fuel the flame of hope. Call it courage, effort, determination, endurance, love, faith. All are signs of spiritual wellness, and all nurture the will to live.

Physical Wellness

Fitness is no longer a craze, but a way of life for many people in the United States. People are running, biking, swimming, and walking in record numbers. Women fill aerobics classes and jazzercise away pounds and inches.

What is physical fitness? Simply put, it is the capacity of the heart, blood vessels, lungs, and muscles to function at optimal efficiency, so daily tasks and recreational activities can be enthusiastically enjoyed. Physically fit individuals have the strength, flexibility, endurance, and cardiorespiratory capacity to continue participating in their normal daily activities.

Keeping Physically Fit with Exercise

When the first measurable snow falls and the ski slopes open, skiers flock to the hills to rediscover the exhilaration of downhill flight. But what they also discover (usually the next morning) is a dull ache in many of the muscles in their arms, legs, and backs. During the spring and summer months, those muscles weren't called into active duty. And now they are suffering from disuse. When you have been ill and inactive, possibly bedridden, for a long time, your body is also suffering from disuse. And the longer you remain inactive, the longer it will take to regain that strength. To avoid those aching muscles, smart skiers work up to the first downhill run with a gradual conditioning program, This type of conditioning program is equally beneficial for people recovering from cancer. Positive results include:

- *Improved prognosis.* A person in good physical condition tolerates therapy better; physical status is an important indicator of successful treatment and improved prognosis.

- *Muscle maintenance.* Muscles shrink in size and strength when not in use. Even a low level of activity improves muscle tone.

- *Speedier recovery.* Surgery and therapy can break down tissues; exercise helps those tissues rebound and minimizes joint deterioration.

- *Mental tonic.* A good way to get your mind off cancer is to get moving. When you're physically engaged in activity, you don't have time to think about negative things.

Physical Conditioning

Simple isometric exercises like the ones at the end of this chapter will help you maintain and increase your range of motion. Because they require little exertion, they can be done in bed. Although you are not moving around to do these exercises, your muscles are still getting a workout by pushing and working against one another.

In their book *Getting Well Again*, O. Carl Simonton, Stephanie Matthews-Simonton, and James L. Creighton prescribe one hour of exercise at least three times a week. For people who are still bedridden, they suggest combining isometric exercises with mental imagery. First, spend five minutes going through the isometric exercise program. For the next ten minutes, use imagery to picture yourself doing a favorite activity—playing tennis, swimming, biking, or just walking in the woods. The activity should be both physically taxing and enjoyable. Alternate between isometrics and imagery until one hour has passed.

If you set aside a specific time for your exercise plan, it will already have become a habit by the time you leave the hospital. Once you are up and around, you can expand your exercise program. The list of 16 light exercises described at the end of this chapter might be used as part of a daily routine when you are first able to be out of bed. They are also especially helpful if you are in a wheelchair. The muscle-strengthening exercises (using light resistance equipment, such as a dumbbell), might be best used as you begin regaining strength.

More important than the form of exercise you choose is its regularity. A regular exercise program is like money in the bank. If you are hospitalized or bedridden again and if your body is in good shape, you will recuperate faster. A combination of walking and jogging for one hour, three times a week, is probably the best all-around exercise. A physical or recreational therapist could help you design a beginning walking program that fits your needs. If you aren't enthusiastic about walking, choose something else you enjoy. And be sure to check with your physician before beginning any exercise program.

Because Malinda enjoys swimming, she joined Encore, a YWCA-sponsored exercise and discussion program for women who have had breast cancer surgery. At Encore, she takes part in both floor and water exercises. After a workout, the women usually eat lunch together and discuss common concerns related to breast cancer and mastectomy.

"I'm the youngest member of this group, and right now the only one who has an active cancer. Actually, I think that makes the others a little nervous. I'm there as a reminder of what they have been through, and of what they could have to go through again," Malinda says.

Jim also chose swimming as his main form of exercise. In addition, he lifts weights to keep his muscles in shape. Debbie plays softball twice a week and tries to walk in between. Lou and Ingvar square dance in addition to taking a daily walk. They all have discovered that exercise can be fun.

Staying active is not only invigorating, but is also a terrific antidote for depression and boredom. By making a commitment to a regular exercise program, you are also making a commitment to living. "My dad says motion is sacred," Bill reiterates, "and he's right. By taking a daily walk up and down the stairs and doing some mild calisthenics in between, I felt pretty good when I left the hospital."

After designing an exercise program to suit your needs, be sure to get your doctor's approval before beginning, then adhere to the following rules to prevent overexertion or injury.

Ten Rules for Safe Exercise

- Start gradually, and have your doctor approve anything unusual or strenuous (jogging, weight lifting, etc.).

- Have someone assist you in doing the exercises, both for your enjoyment and your safety. This is particularly important when you are first getting out of bed.

- If you get tired or your muscles feel sore, stop and rest.

- Avoid eating for at least one hour before exercise because it can add stress and increase blood pressure.

- Don't exercise if you have a cold, cough, flu, etc. Wait until you feel better.

- Never strain, hold your breath, or allow yourself to get red in the face. This puts excess burden on the heart and circulatory system.

- Keep a slow and steady pace. Don't hurry. The heart is a muscle too and gets tired. Rest and start again.

- Try to repeat each exercise three to five times at first. Gradually increase to 10 or 20 repetitions.

- Work for good posture. Slumping causes muscle strain and puts an extra workload on the heart.

- Be regular. One hour three times a week is ideal, but do what you can, when you can, depending on your other daily activities.

Exercise As a Mental Stimulus

Besides providing physical conditioning, exercise can also be a good mental tonic. Anyone who has spent even a few days sick in bed is aware of how quickly the body weakens when immobile. And often the spirit weakens at the same time. Activity is actually an antidote for depression, and sometimes exercising makes more sense than taking medication. As a stress reliever, a brisk walk may be more beneficial than a tranquilizer.

When you exercise, you are in control. You take charge of your schedule, decide what to do, and how long you will do it. Along with the physical accomplishment, you end up feeling more in charge of your life. A healthier body contributes to a healthier mind. Cancer creates stress. Without finding ways to diminish that stress, it is difficult to achieve both physical and mental well being. If people are able to reduce stress in addition to staying active right up to the top of their physical abilities, they feel more self-sufficient, have a stronger sense of self-worth, and hopefully minimize depression.

Keeping active encompasses every part of daily living, starting from the simplest of tasks, like getting out of bed, to devising and carrying out a vigorous exercise plan. The person with cancer must discover a comfortable program somewhere between these two extremes.

Strategies for Keeping Active

After her recurrence, Malinda had radiation in the morning and then took a nap before work. "I would get mad at myself for having to take a nap. I wanted to continue doing things the way I used to. I wanted everything to be normal." But cancer and its treatment force people to reassess what is "normal" in their lives. And like it or not, much of our self-esteem is tied to the simple, daily things we are accustomed to doing. Malinda's nap time forced her to give up part of her daily routine. And that meant letting the housework slide.

Malinda began to feel like she wasn't doing her part anymore. She started feeling dependent. Her feelings of dependence became even more pronounced when she was forced to ask for help. During chemotherapy, driving was out of the question.

Malinda had to rely on the help of others. She says, "I felt like an invalid asking someone to drive me to treatment and then wait around and drive me home. I quickly realized how demoralizing it is to be dependent."

At this point, Malinda was at yet another crossroad in her struggle between controlling cancer and letting cancer control her. Would she allow herself to become dependent, or would she adjust her lifestyle to preserve as much independence as possible? "I had to admit that I needed help with some things. But I was determined to hold onto my independence in every way possible. I was learning what it felt like to be an invalid. And I didn't want that to be a permanent condition."

Conserving Personal Energy

The key to conserving personal energy is to work smarter, not harder. If achieving maximum independence is your goal, try the following suggestions:

Lower your personal standards.

Trying to keep up at your old pace can only lead to frustration. If you are accustomed to keeping a spotless house, lower your standards to simply having an uncluttered house. If you mow the lawn once a week, settle on twice a month. Stop ironing clothes, and either take them to the dry cleaner or hang shirts up straight out of the dryer. Superman or Superwoman no longer has a place in your home.

Start each day with a priority list.

Before going to bed, make a list of what you hope to do the next day. Start with things that *must* be done:

- Get out of bed.
- Eat breakfast.
- Go to Dr. appointment.
- Go for radiation treatments, etc.

After the *musts* come the *maybes*:

- Do the laundry.
- Wash the dishes.
- Go to the store
- Pay the bills.

Finish your list with things that *would be nice*:

- Correspondence.
- Clean the bathroom.
- Wash the car.
- Rake leaves, etc.

By starting with a list, you can avoid wasting time on unimportant activities at the expense of those that are important. Make sure that among the "musts" is at least one activity that is purely for your benefit. Set aside an hour for a favorite television show, a trip to the library, or lunch with a friend. At day's end, give yourself points for every task accomplished. There may be days, particularly right after treatment, when just getting out of bed, getting dressed, and eating a meal are three major accomplishments for that day. Pat yourself on the back for doing all three.

Balance activity and rest.

"I'm finally learning how to relax," admits Jim, after years of being a workaholic. "One important thing I have learned to do is quit working before I start feeling tired. Now I can stop at two or three in the afternoon. I can actually drop the rake with leaves still on the ground." Knowing when to stop can mean the difference between a good day and a tiring day. Analyze your day and pace yourself so the work is equal to your activity level. Do heavier tasks (house painting) when energy is high, and save lighter tasks (correspondence, bill paying) for rest times.

Strive to simplify.

The less you have to contend with, the more you can get done. The following suggestions may prove helpful:

- Eliminate depressing, dust-collecting clutter than can slow you down and wear you out, physically and mentally. Put all

155

nonessential items in boxes and store them in an attic, sell them at a garage sale, or give them to charity.

- Empty closets and drawers of all clothes you don't wear and ask someone to take them to Goodwill for you. Learn to say no to time-wasting, nonproductive activities. When you felt better, it was easy to volunteer for church bazaars or school projects. Now you need all your energy to get well.

When all else fails, ask for help.

Sometimes, you know you're not going to feel better unless a particular project is done. But you just don't have the energy to do it. This is where family and friends can help. Take the big step and ask someone to scrub your floors, mow your lawn, or clean your refrigerator.

Each of us can identify at least one thing about our environment that drives us nuts. Malinda went crazy if her ironing piled up or if her clothes didn't look just right. For Jim, looking at an unkempt yard was almost unbearable. Malinda needed to ask her friend Evie to help with the ironing and run to the dry cleaners once a week. Jim's son agreed to pick up the slack and help keep the yard neat. By learning to ask others for help, both Malinda and Jim were able to control those important environmental concerns.

Self-Help Strategies for Daily Activities

"I do it myself," exclaims the toddler as he takes his first steps toward a lifetime of independence. We all want to do it without help if we can. People with cancer generally recover faster and feel more responsible for their recovery when they continue to perform most of their regular daily activities. Some of the benefits of continued activity include the following:

• Increased ability to perform tasks.

• Improved muscle tone.

• Improved range of motion.

• Satisfaction of setting and completing goals.

By keeping a Self-Care Progress Record similar to the example at the end of this chapter, you have evidence of daily progress. Mastery of a new activity enhances self-esteem and fuels the will to live.

Self-Help Assistive Devices

Assistive devices such as cups with lids or grab bars next to a tub compensate for loss of function. Most can be obtained from medical and surgical supply stores or by mail order from companies specializing in self-help devices.

For eating and drinking:

• Use a cup with a lid prevents spilling.

• Drink from a Wonder-Flow vacuum cup even if you are lying flat on your back.

• Use stretch knit coasters to compensate for a weak grasp.

• When in bed, use a wedge-shaped cushion behind your back and a tray with legs.

For independent bathing:

• Install grab bars next to the tub.

• Use a bath seat for sitting in the tub.

• Use a portable shower head and a bath seat so you can take a shower without standing up.

• Use a raised toilet seat to make it easier to stand up.

For independent dressing:

- Do as much as possible while seated in an arm chair.

- Put your weak arm or leg in your clothing first.

- Take your strong arm or leg out of your clothing first when you are undressing.

- Buy an attractive, loose-fitting lounge coat if you are not wearing street clothes yet.

For accomplishing housework:

- Write out a weekly plan for major tasks and make sure you do only one major task per day (laundry, shopping, cleaning, ironing, etc.)

- Use comforters instead of bedspreads on beds. Just pull them up and the bed is made!

For simplifying meal preparation:
- During peak energy times, make double-size meals and freeze part of them for later use.

- Plan menus ahead of time and choose things that can be put together easily (casseroles, TV dinners, hot dogs, hamburgers, canned spaghetti, or creamed soups). Include family members in planning and preparation.

- Let someone else do the cooking.

- Accept gifts of food and freeze them for later use.

- Use paper plates and cups whenever possible.

- Use a crock pot for easy, one-pot meals that cook while you rest.

- Order food from a favorite restaurant and bring it home to eat.

Reducing Stress and Tension

The phone is ringing. The baby is crying. The dog is barking. The pan on the stove is boiling over. Life's everyday stresses can send people over the edge. The new stresses associated with cancer can exacerbate that plunge. What can you do about it?

What Is Stress Anyway?

Stress is a normal response to the demands of everyday life. It's a form of energy, and in itself it's neither bad nor good. Weddings can produce stress. Giving a holiday party brings on stress. But the response doesn't necessarily have to be negative. The stress can provide us with extra energy to accomplish the many things necessary during these times.

Of course, stress occurs during bad times too. The obvious stress of encountering a brown bear in the thick of a forest brings out our primitive "fight-or-flight" reflex. The heart speeds up. Muscles get tense. We start to breathe heavily and the blood rushes to our arms and legs. Our body is giving us a choice—either fight or get away fast! In today's world, most of life's problems cannot be solved by fighting or running away. Instead of expending the energy brought on by the "fight-or-flight" reflex, our bodies internalize the stress. As a result, this prolonged, unrelieved stress creates a variety of physical symptoms, including high blood pressure, headaches, or dizziness.

If stress can bring on headaches and backaches, what other physical ailments can it cause? This question is one of the most hotly debated items in medicine.

Are Stress and Disease Related?

Dr. Hans Selye, who has written more than 38 books on the subject of stress, including the popular *Stress Without Distress*, first started studying the link between stress and disease in the 1920s. He believes that stress is involved in all human illness.

Most experts agree that stress lowers the body's ability to fight off illness.

When Malinda returned from Louisiana after visiting her husband, her back was aching. She soon discovered that the cancer had metastasized to her bones. She partially blames the ongoing stress of her floundering marriage for her physical setback. "My husband moved down south, and I agreed to go visit him in July. It was our six-year wedding anniversary, and he wanted us to be together. Talking about my cancer always causes problems, so I just kept my mouth shut and did what he wanted to do. It's hard to pretend you're healthy and everything is okay when it isn't. It was stressful for me, to say the least. Once I learned the results of my bone scan, I was angry with myself for taking the trip. I know the stress of the trip didn't cause the cancer to return. But I'm sure it didn't help either. And it did contribute to the symptoms."

Individuals react to stress differently, based on their personalities. Studies have even been done attempting to identify "cancer-prone" personality types. Without solid evidence, this seems to be a cruel hoax—assigning blame to the person with the disease. The results of these studies are far from conclusive. And for the person with cancer, theories on at-risk personality types are of no value. What is important now is learning new coping skills to help reduce stress.

Researchers at Massachusetts General Hospital (Weisman, Worden, Sobel) studying cancer patients found that those who coped best were not necessarily those with the most favorable physical prognosis. But they did have the following characteristics in common:

- *Optimism.* They expected positive change was possible.

- *Practicality.* They could assess what solutions were feasible.

- *Flexibility.* They weren't rigid in their approach.

- *Resourcefulness.* They looked for support and additional information.

Bertrand Russell wrote: "It is not the experience that happens to you. It is what you do with the experience that happens to you." Stress is not the event of having cancer. Stress is the individual's inner feelings about that event and the subsequent reactions based on those feelings. Those reactions can change the level of hormones secreted from the adrenal glands. These hormones, in turn, affect responses of the immune system.

How a person copes with stress is the most important factor in determining how that stress will affect the immune system. No one knows the extent to which this mind-body connection affects the course of an illness. No tests or measurement tools are currently available that would offer much data. But hundreds of case histories suggest that we shouldn't disregard the connection.

Fifteen Proven Ways to Reduce Stress

1. *Get enough exercise.* Exercise is a valuable method of letting off steam. In addition, physical activity helps relieve frustration and boredom, lessens aggressive feelings, and helps control weight.

    Exercise has an added benefit. It helps you develop a sense of self-confidence and accomplishment. Last week you could only walk to the corner. Today you can make it around the block. Daily exercise can give you a surge of energy as well as a happier outlook.

2. *Eat properly.* When you are under stress, your nutritional needs increase. Your body uses food faster. You need protein, vitamins, and minerals to repair damage caused by stress. People with cancer get a double benefit from eating properly. A good diet rebuilds the cells damaged by treatment and also helps reduce stress.

3. *Develop the leisure activities you enjoy.* Remember the adage "Idle hands are the devil's workshop"? If you drop many of your old hobbies because thoughts of cancer have you immobilized, stress is bound to build up. Force yourself to get back in the swing of things. Can't think of anything? Here are some suggestions:

—Bake a cake.	—Start a journal.
—Build a doghouse.	—Join a new club.
—Paint a picture.	—Sew a new outfit.
—Take a walk.	—Take in a movie.
—Put in new rose bushes.	—Collect stamps or rocks
—Cook a gourmet dinner.	—Visit an old friend.

The list is endless. Activity takes your mind off your illness. And it's fun!

4. *Watch your self-talk.* Who do you talk to most every day? Yourself! And if you start paying attention, you'll probably be surprised at how many negative messages you're giving yourself. Are you saying things like "This is awful. I'll never make it," or "I shouldn't have to put up with this," or "I look so awful; I'm sure no one wants to be with me." These negative thoughts create tension. By making a conscious choice to be encouraging rather than discouraging, you can eliminate that tension. Whenever you catch yourself saying, "I can't. I won't. I shouldn't," think of the railroad engine in the children's story, *The Little Engine That Could.* All the way up that steep hill, the little engine chanted "I think I can, I think I can." And so it was.

At the end of the day, give yourself a positive pep talk. Add up all the things you've done right and compliment yourself. Drop the word "should" from your vocabulary and substitute "could" or "want to."

5. *Get involved in something larger than yourself.* Reaching out to help others takes the focus off you and reduces the stress caused by brooding. Most people with cancer speak of their need to do something for others. For this reason, people-helping-people programs such as Reach to Recovery and Cansurmount always have ready volunteers. When you immerse yourself in a cause, whether it is religious, political, or cancer related, it takes the steam out of your worries and gives you a gratifying feeling of having done something for others.

6. *Talk it out.* Bottling up worries and fears only builds up tension. Someone once said that a good friend is worth a hundred psychiatrists. Confide in someone you respect and trust—your husband or wife, father or mother, a good friend, your clergyperson, your family physician, a teacher, or a school counselor. Talking about problems won't solve them. But just having the conversation will reduce stress. Seek professional assistance if necessary. You're worth it.

7. *Develop your problem-solving skills.* The first step in problem solving is to clearly identify the problem. Write it down so it's clear in your mind. Are there any facts you're missing? Are you making assumptions that may not be true? What would happen if you did nothing? After getting the necessary facts, list your options. Think of at least four things you could do to solve your problem. List the pros and cons of each. After weighing your options, choose a plan. Then list the necessary steps to carry that plan through to completion. Give yourself a deadline. Then act. Just having a plan to solve the problem can make you feel better and reduce your stress.

8. *Learn to pace yourself.* Stop before you get tired. When you're feeling strong, don't waste time sitting around. But when your energy starts to fade, take a break. At the end of

the day, you want to feel you've accomplished something, but not at the expense of your mental or physical health.

9. *Learn to say no.* There is a difference between doing things for others and having others take advantage of you. If you believe someone or some group is making an unreasonable request, feel free to say no without making excuses. Stick to your word without feeling guilty.

10. *Give in occasionally.* Not every argument is worth winning. People learning to live with cancer often feel frustrated because they're no longer able to control their own fate. This frustration can result in frequent quarrels with others. But trying to control others may only make them more defensive and cause more stress. There are two sides to every issue. It's easier on your system to yield once in a while. If you do, you'll find others will too.

11. *Focus on the positive.* If you suffer a setback, take stock of your achievements to restore self-confidence. In *Stress Without Distress*, Selye suggests you also "try to keep your mind on pleasant aspects of life and on actions that can improve your situation. Try to forget everything that is irrevocably ugly or painful."

12. *Take one thing at a time.* "Divide and conquer" is valuable advice on days when everything seems overwhelming. If you divide up the tasks and simply take one at a time (pitching into the most urgent ones first), they will miraculously disappear. You'll get more done with less hassle when you concentrate on each job as it comes.

13. *Eliminate Superman or Superwoman from your life.* You may have been "doing it all" before, but there is no room for perfectionism now. List your priorities, choose the things you must do yourself, and then delegate the rest. Family and friends are secretly wondering what they can do for you. So tell them!

14. *Have a good laugh at least once a day.* In his book *Anatomy of an Illness*, Norman Cousins popularized the theory of laughter as a healing force. Scientists have shown that laughter triggers the brain to release chemicals called endorphins. The endorphins are capable of blocking pain and giving us a sense of well being.

Go see a whimsical movie. Listen to a favorite comedian on tape. Read the comic pages in the newspaper daily. Cut out your favorites and start a bulletin board. Tack up your favorite jokes, funny pictures, or humorous things that have happened to you. Sharing a good laugh with a friend is an inexpensive and healing prescription.

15. *Get adequate sleep.* Any parent who has been up with a baby all night will admit to feeling stressed the next day. Often people with cancer take their worries to bed with them. They toss and turn as they ponder the "what ifs" of their life. Adopt a policy of leaving your worries outside the bedroom door. Your bed is for sleeping.

In addition, make sure you're tired before you go to bed. You can do this by getting adequate exercise during the day, avoiding caffeine, and perhaps having a warm bath or warm drink before bed.

If you don't sleep well for a long period of time (weeks), or if you feel tired every morning, see your doctor. It could be a sign of clinical depression.

Relaxation—The Ultimate Stress Reducer

Relaxation means different things to different people. And for many people, relaxation doesn't come naturally. The stresses brought on by cancer are often so intense that people need to learn new relaxation techniques and practice them regularly. Three relaxation skills that are often helpful are meditation, visual imagery, and acupressure.

Meditation

Dr. Herbert Benson, while doing research on stress at Harvard Medical School, Boston, concentrated on a method called the "relaxation response." His method used some of the mechanics of ancient meditation, but he eliminated the religious or cultic overtones. The relaxation response is a way of reducing anxiety without drugs. The mechanics include four elements:

- *A quiet environment.* Find a quiet place where you will not be disturbed. Eliminate all distractions. Background noise may prevent the proper response.

- *A passive attitude.* By trying to force the relaxation response, you may prevent it from occurring at all. The purpose of the response is to relax, so be completely passive. Disregard distracting thoughts that enter your mind.

- *A comfortable position.* Sit in a comfortable chair in as restful a position as possible. The purpose is to keep muscular effort to a minimum, so the head and arms should be supported. Remove your shoes and prop up your feet several inches. Loosen all tight-fitting clothing. Sitting is probably better than lying down because you don't want to fall asleep.

- *Mentally focus on a single word or sound.* Repeat a single-syllable sound or word, sometimes called a mantra, silently or in a low, gentle tone. Any word will work, but because of its simplicity and neutrality, the word "one" is suggested.

Once you have these four elements in place, it is possible to elicit the relaxation response by progressively relaxing your muscles and establishing a rhythmic breathing pattern. As you concentrate on each muscle group, breathe in through your nose, then say "one" silently to yourself as you breathe out. As you continue breathing and repeating the mantra, concentrate on your body and areas where you feel muscle tightness. The next time you breathe, eliminate the tightness in that area. When you feel your body is totally relaxed, eliminate all thoughts and concentrate on breathing. When other thoughts enter your mind, disregard them. Continue this practice for 20 minutes. You may open your eyes to check the time, but do not use an alarm. When you finish, sit quietly for several minutes with your eyes closed. Tell yourself to remain calm and feel refreshed when you get up and resume your activities. Open your eyes and rest a bit longer.

Don't expect great things to happen at once. Meditation improves with practice. In the beginning, you may only find it serves as a restful interval. Your mind may wander often, and it may be difficult to remain fixed on your chosen word. But with practice, you should reach a point where you can detach yourself from your physical surroundings and keep your mind free of distractions. Many people have found immense satisfaction from a daily program of relaxation therapy.

At the end of this chapter is a script of a deep breathing exercise for practicing meditation. It can be used most successfully by recording the words on tape, then playing them back while listening to your favorite soothing music. Many commercially available tapes also facilitate the relaxation response. By checking around in your area, you should be able to find more material. In Chapter 7, Identifying Support Systems and Resources, you will find a list of companies that produce tape recordings of relaxation and imagery.

Visual Imagery

Once you have mastered the deep breathing techniques and are able to move easily into a meditative state, visual imagery can be another very effective relaxation technique. You simply visualize a color, a scene, or a place that you find extremely relaxing. This could be a warm beach or a cool meadow. You could be floating on a cloud or surrounded by a bright light. Because visualizations are totally personal, you are free to let your mind explore the images that are most comfortable for you.

At the end of this chapter is a script for a visualization exercise that invites you to find your own peaceful place. Again, it will probably be most effective if you slowly record the script, allowing for pauses where the script indicates, then playing it back while also listening to soothing music.

Acupressure

Acupressure is a more convenient form of acupuncture, a treatment method developed in China more than 2000 years ago for the relief of pain. Acupressure techniques, which can induce relaxation and relieve stress, are easy to learn and can be self-administered. At the end of this chapter, you will find a more complete description of acupressure with some illustrations to help get you started.

Uncertainty—The Ultimate Stress

Bertrand Russell once said, "To teach men how to live without certainty, and yet without being paralyzed by hesitation, is perhaps the chief thing philosophy can still do."

People with cancer are always waiting for the other shoe to drop. Every new ache or pain paralyzes them with fear. "It's like running a red light and looking in the rear view mirror to see if a cop is chasing you," Bill says. "You want to believe you've made it through safely. Most likely you have. But there's always that chance." Bill knows the pull of uncertainty. When he had been in remission five years, his doctors started cautiously using the word "cured." Bill wanted to believe them. After 10 years, he was finally ready to believe it. And then an elevated blood marker once again reminded Bill of the cop that had been chasing him all those years.

The statistics on survival for Bill's type of testicular cancer are still excellent. Despite his recurrence, Bill is now free of cancer and can expect to remain in remission for years. But he doesn't include the word "cure" in his vocabulary anymore. "I don't think any of us can realistically use the word cured," Bill says. "We know we don't have cancer right now. But we can never be sure that it won't return."

For Malinda, the uncertainty is not whether the cancer will return. Instead, she wonders how long it can be controlled. "I know the odds," she says philosophically. "Even though I want to be one of the 3 percent with this type of cancer who make it, I have to face the fact that maybe I won't." How does she do that? "One day at a time," she says. "I know that sounds trite, but it is the healthiest approach to take. I get so mad at these people who waste time worrying or feeling sorry for themselves. If you feel good today, don't worry about tomorrow. Get out there and make the most of it."

Cancer does not necessarily make life more uncertain. It simply magnifies the uncertainty of life.

Suggested Reading

To learn more about topics discussed in Chapter 4, the following reading material is recommended:

Bell, Lorna, R.N., and Eudora Seyfer. *Gentle Yoga: A Guide to Gentle Exercise.* Berkeley, CA: Celestial Arts, 1987.

Benson, Herbert, and Miriam Z. Klipper. *The Relaxation Response.* New York: Avon, 1976. Explains relaxation and provides techniques.

Carty, Amy. *Positive Visualizations: For People with Cancer and Those who Love Them.* Birchard Books, RR2, Box 179, Washington Mt. Rd., Lee, MA 01038, 1992.

Gawain, Shakti. *Creative Visualization.* New York: Bantam Books, 1982. Help in understanding visualization and affirmations.

Lerner, Helene. *Stress Breakers.* Minneapolis: Comp Care, 1989.

Meichenbaum, Dr. Donald. *Coping With Stress.* New York: Facts on File, 1983.

Self Care Catalog and Journal. 349 Healdsburg Avenue, Healdsburg, CA 94558 (products and articles about health and fitness, including massage, exercise, stress reduction)

Slaby, Andrew E. *60 Ways To Make Stress Work For You.* New York: Bantam Books, 1991.

Isometric Exercises

**While lying down and looking straight ahead,
do the following:**

- Place the heel of your right hand on your forehead and push your forehead against your hand.

- Place the palm of your right hand against the back of your head and push your head backward against the force of your hand.

- Place the palm of your right hand against the right side of your head and push your head to the right, resisting the pressure of your hand.

- Clench your teeth, raise your head slightly, and forcefully pull the corners of your mouth outward and down.

While in a sitting position, do the following:

- Put the palms of your hands together and forcefully push them against each other.

- Clasp your hands together, and then try to forcefully pull them apart.

Sixteen Light Exercises

Remember: Exercise can relax you, improve your circulation, help with lung expansion, and improve the quality of sleep. Start any exercise program slowly and easily.

You may do the following exercises either standing or sitting.

1. Put your hands on the arms of your chair or in your lap. Pull your shoulder blades together as you breathe in deeply. Relax and slowly exhale.

2. Shrug your shoulders up, and then slowly let them down. Then completely relax.

3. Place your hands on the arm or the seat of a chair. Push with your hands as if to lift yourself up out of the chair. Do not push with your feet.

4. Squeeze your buttocks tightly together. Count to five. Then relax. Keep breathing; don't hold your breath.

5. Put your right hand on your left knee and try to lift your knee up, but press so hard with your hand that you can't actually lift it. Relax. Repeat with your other leg.

6. Lift your arms out in front of your face and up over your head, keeping your elbows straight. Do one arm at a time. If this is comfortable, do both arms together and reach for the ceiling.

7. Lift your arms out to your sides and up over your head. Then do one arm at a time.

8. Straighten your knees as much as possible, one at a time. Then do both knees at the same time.

9. Press your heels into the floor as if to lift yourself out of your chair.

10. Dig your heels into the floor as if to dig a hole.

11. Place your right hand on your right shoulder, and your left hand on your left shoulder. Move your elbows in circles.

12. Cross your arms in front of your chest. Then move them back as if to touch your elbows behind your back.

13. Grab the arm of your chair and attempt to bend your elbow. Relax. You may also this exercise by holding an object weighing 5 pounds or less and lifting it to your shoulder by bending your elbow.

14. Place your hands together in front of your chest, as if in prayer. Straighten your fingers as much as possible. Push your hands together. Relax.

15. Fold your hands together. Try to pull them apart.

16. Lift your foot slightly off the floor. Point your toes, first up, then down. Then make circles with your foot.

Each exercise produces tension for a brief period of time (five to ten seconds) without a great deal of physical exertion. "No movement" exercises like these develop strength with a minimum of time and equipment. Start by doing each exercise five times and gradually increase to ten times. These can be done once or twice daily, energy permitting. Hold each exercise for a count of ten.

Self-Care Progress Record

Goal: To help you assess your energy output and your independence in daily living skills. Post this where you can easily check off the completed activity daily.

	S	M	T	W	Th	F	S
I got out of bed before noon.							
I bathed/showered without help.							
I dressed myself without help.							
I made breakfast.							
I ate breakfast at the table.							
I exercised today.							
I fixed lunch/dinner.							
I ate lunch/dinner at the table.							
I went out of the house today.							
I did a recreational activity today.							

* Adapted from a questionnaire from the Physical Therapy Department, North Memorial Medical Center, Minneapolis, MN

Fill in boxes below with things you would have liked to do each day but did not or could not.

Sun.	
Mon.	
Tues.	
Wed.	
Thur.	
Fri.	
Sat.	

Script for Deep Breathing Exercise

Everything we do or think is reflected in our breathing. A happy, relaxed person breathes with a calm, regulated rhythm. A stressed, angry, or depressed person's breathing becomes shallow, uneven, and spasmodic. To demonstrate this concept, spend the next 30 seconds concentrating on an item of jewelry that you or someone else is wearing. It could be a ring, an earring, a bracelet, a watch, a pin. When the 30 seconds are up, do you notice a change in your breathing as a result of concentrating on this object? Deep breathing increases the supply of oxygen to the brain. Because of this, many people feel an energy boost after even a brief deep breathing exercise.

Before engaging in any deep breathing exercise, it's important to know a few general rules about deep breathing.

- Always breathe in through the nose. People who practice yoga believe the mouth is for eating and talking only. The nose has a built-in warming and filtering system to cleanse the air before it reaches the lungs.

- Success takes practice. Each time you participate in a deep-breathing exercise, either alone or with a group, you will get more proficient at it. Don't worry about achieving a deep level of relaxation first time around. Instead, maintain a passive attitude and let relaxation come on its own time schedule.

- Practice with an empty stomach.

Find a comfortable position where the spine is straight, feet and arms are at rest, and eyes are closed. Then listen to your pre-recorded version of the following script.

Script

These moments are yours. They are dedicated to your health and well-being. During this time, you have nowhere to go and nothing to do. Your only goal is to become aware of your breathing and to center on your own inner strength. The problems of the day will wait for you. For now, your focus is inward toward the very center of your body.

(Pause)

Inhale slowly through your nose, filling the abdomen as if blowing up a balloon between your waist and your thighs. Picture your ribs stretching outward as your middle chest fills. Then fill your upper lungs until you feel them stretching up to your shoulders. Hold that breath and think of the word "one." When you feel the need to exhale, continue to think of the word "one" as you let the breath out through your nose, starting at your shoulders and feeling it sink like an elevator down through your upper lungs, slowly deflating your middle chest and pulling your ribs back into place, then finally breathing out all the air in the balloon inside your abdomen.

(Pause)

As you slowly take in your next breath, become aware of the muscles in your body. Start at your feet and work up to your face, consciously letting go of any tension still remaining in any spot. Concentrate on eliminating all muscle tension in your body as you fill your lungs once more. As you begin to exhale, once again concentrate on the word "one." Repeat the word as often as you like, then feel the elevator sink once more, starting at your shoulders, moving slowly through your upper lungs, down to your middle chest, and finally deflating the balloon in your abdomen.

(Pause)

As you slowly begin to take in the final breath of this exercise, imagine the air you are taking into your lungs is filled with calmness. Feel the warm calmness fill the balloon, then ride the elevator up through your middle chest, expanding your ribs and finally filling your upper lungs with serenity all the way to your shoulders. As you begin to exhale, again think of the word "one." Repeat the word "one" as you try to eliminate any other word or thought from your mind. Now slowly exhale this last breath.

(Pause)

Begin to reacquaint yourself with your surroundings. Open your eyes and smile. Keep this pleasant feeling with you as you go about your day.

Script for Guided Visualization

Guided imagery works best when you design your own environment instead of entering an environment of someone else's design. That environment can be a special place that already exists for you, a place you have always wanted to go, or a place that exists only in your imagination. Only one criteria exists for this "peaceful place": it must satisfy your ideal concept of relaxation, tranquility, and safety. Keeping that in mind, you can create this peaceful place exactly as you wish.

Find a comfortable position where the spine is straight and feet and arms are at rest. To center yourself, focus on a spot on the ceiling for a few seconds, then slowly lower your head and at the same time close your eyes. Be silent for a moment, clearing your mind of all images and thoughts. While listening to your favorite soothing music, play back your prerecorded version of the following script.

Script

These moments are yours. They are dedicated to your health and well being. During this time, you have nowhere to go and nothing to do. Your only goal is to pay attention to your breath and center on your own inner strength. The problems of this day will wait for you. For now, your focus is inward toward the very center of your body.

(Pause)

Breathe in deeply, paying close attention to your breath, and fill your insides with warm, cleansing air. If thoughts or pictures enter your mind, imagine a giant television screen in front of you. Place all bothersome thoughts on the giant television screen, then mentally reach up and turn the set off. The screen is blank and the sound is gone. Your mind is empty except for the sound of your breath. Breathe deeply and pay attention only to your breath.

(Pause)

Continue your deep breathing as a dot appears on your screen and slowly grows until it is an enormous hot air balloon, fully inflated with the vivid colors of a rainbow. The balloon floats toward you now and waits while you climb in the wicker basket, then lifts off to take you to your peaceful place. As you float upward through the clouds, past the birds, you look down on the earth and begin to picture your destination, the place where you will eventually land. That destination is your peaceful place, a sanctuary where you feel comfortable, pleasant, and safe. It could be a grassy meadow or a towering mountaintop . . . in the cool of a forest or the open warmth of a prairie field. You could come to rest beside the waters of a cool stream, a placid lake, or the pounding surf. You may end up in a favorite country . . . a favorite city . . . in a favorite building . . . in a favorite room . . . or in a place that is totally a creation of your own imagination. You know exactly where you are headed by now, and your balloon is about to land at that peaceful place. You see it in the distance and watch it moving closer. Your balloon drifts slowly toward earth and gently touches down. You look around for a moment, then step out and walk to your favorite part of this peaceful place. Get comfortable now and explore your environment for a moment, noting the visual details . . . the sounds . . . the smells . . . the feel of where you are seated.

(Pause)

Now do whatever is necessary to make this place more home-like and comfortable for you. If you are outdoors, you may wish to create a shelter for yourself. If you are indoors, you could prepare your favorite food . . . your favorite drink . . . get involved in an activity that gives you pleasure and comfort. Relax and enjoy the sights, the sounds, the smells, the taste . . . of this peaceful place that is yours and yours alone. Memorize this place and know you can and will return to it whenever your mind needs peace and rest.

(Pause)

Your balloon is waiting to take you back to reality. Climb in and feel yourself floating upward through space, over the lands that separate your peaceful place from the reality of this day. As you float through the clouds and back down to earth, hold onto the peacefulness, tranquility, and absolute safety of where you have been.

(Allow a few moments of silence)

You watch the colorful rainbow-colored balloon slowly disappear into the distance until it is only a small dot on your screen. Now begin to reacquaint yourself with your surroundings. Open your eyes—and smile. Keep this pleasant feeling with you as you go about your day.

Use of Acupressure to Reduce Stress

Acupressure techniques are easy to learn and can be self-administered. If a point can be found on both sides of the body (for instance, on the left and right hand or left and right feet), it tends to be more effective to use both during one session. Be sure to follow timing instructions, as timing makes a difference in the outcome. Treatments can be repeated several times per day. Take a moment before you begin to center your thoughts as you receive or give a treatment.

Once you locate the point, press with your fingertip, giving a slightly rotating motion for the prescribed length of time. Most of the time the point will be tender while you press. This is normal. Press firmly, but gently. If you seem to have trouble finding the point but have found a tender area in the general vicinity, go ahead. Points are areas of energy and have the capacity to move an inch or two.

#1, LI 4 The Aspirin Point (Do not use during pregnancy)
Often referred to as the aspirin point of Chinese medicine, this technique can be used for headaches, to lift the spirit, or revitalize energy. Its strong influence makes it one of the four important gates or pillars of acupressure.
Location: In the valley between thumb and first finger.
Duration: Press for about 60 seconds.

#2, HT 7 Shen Ment
Shen refers to the spirit and Ment means gate. The Spirit Gate quiets the spirit, helps insomnia, calms a racing heart, and reduces palpitations. This exercise calms the mind and body.
Location: On the inside of the wrist, at the wrist crease, at the end of the bone.
Duration: Press for 15-30 seconds.

#3, PC 6 The Inner Pass

Similar to HT 7, this point has a calming, quieting effect on the body, mind, and spirit. It works well for nervousness and is best used in conjunction with HT 7.

Location: Two inches above inside of wrist, between the two muscle sinews.

Duration: Press for 15-30 seconds.

#4, GB 14 Yang White

This is especially good for headaches, tension, and anxiety.

Location: On the forehead, 1 inch above the middle of the eyebrows.

Duration: Press for 30 seconds.

(Adapted from material supplied by Bev Jagiello, Certified Acupressurist, St. Paul, Minnesota.)

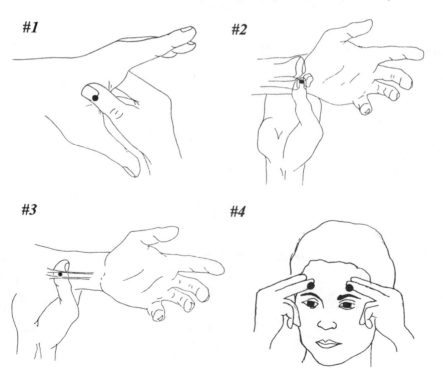

#1 **#2**

#3 **#4**

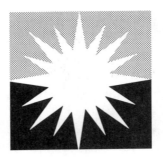

"The careful balance between

silence and words,

withdrawal and involvement,

distance and closeness,

solitude and community

forms the basis of . . . life

and should therefore

be the subject of our

most personal attention."

Henri J. M. Nouwen
Out of Solitude

CHAPTER FIVE

Communicating Concerns and Feelings About Cancer

Above the crib in many babies' rooms hangs a brightly colored mobile. The mobile is suspended from a hook by a series of delicate bars and strings. Several colorful objects designed to attract the baby's eye dangle from the strings. If left untouched, the mobile hangs perfectly still with all pieces balanced. Only when you touch it do you realize how delicate that balance really is. A tiny fist making contact with one of the objects sets them all dancing wildly about. Suddenly, the pieces bounce around uncontrollably, twisting and turning in an attempt to reestablish some sort of equilibrium.

Identifying and Understanding Feelings

When cancer becomes part of a family's life, it enters like a giant fist striking the family's well-balanced mobile. Although the fist has really hit only one object, its rippling effect is felt by all. Family members are jarred out of their comfortable spots. Spinning around in circles with no apparent direction, they meet and clash with one another. Often it has been years since they shared any real feelings. But before this family's mobile comes to rest, they will probably all experience six major emotions: shock or disbelief, anger, denial, sadness or depression, uncertainty, and fear.

All of these feelings are reflections of a person's response to loss and change. From the moment the word "cancer" is spoken, life changes. After feeling safe and secure for so many years, it is both frightening and infuriating to come face to face with mortality.

Shock and Disbelief

Hearing the news that you have diabetes or heart disease is upsetting or disquieting. But hearing you have cancer can be paralyzing. Why? Because cancer has a bad reputation. Many people consider it a deadly, spreading, fatal disease, so disbelief is an understandable reaction to the diagnosis. Cancer is a disease that will strike someone else, not me.

Surprisingly, disbelief can actually serve a useful purpose, since it provides a calming, numbing effect that softens the harsh news. While insulated from the reality of the diagnosis, the person with cancer has an opportunity to begin adjusting to a major life change.

Anger

How dare this happen? I won't allow it. It isn't fair. Why me? Why now? I don't deserve it. All these reactions are examples of expressed anger. Anger at the cancer. Anger at God for letting it happen. Anger at friends and loved ones who are still healthy reminders of the way life used to be.

Anger is a mask to cover other feelings that are more difficult to express. To admit you're hurting or afraid means acknowledging that you are vulnerable. Expressing anger is easier than admitting helplessness. Anger also sometimes disguises feelings of panic. By denying the disease or lashing out in anger, people with cancer can buy some time to let the debilitating panic they are feeling subside.

When a child darts out into a busy street, the mother's reaction is an example of how anger can be a cover for other more realistic feelings. Afraid that her child will be hurt, she panics. She is worried about the child's safety, realizing that at that moment, she is helpless against oncoming cars. In an instant, she comes face to face with her child's mortality. Simultaneously, she experiences fear, panic, worry, and a sense of helplessness. How does she react? With anger.

A typical mother might scream in anger and maybe swat the child's bottom. Anger is the swiftest and easiest response. For the moment, it takes precedence over all her other emotions. Because people often experience delays in getting their cancer accurately diagnosed, their anger may be directed at the medical community. Both Malinda and Lothair posed the question, "Would that six weeks or one month have made a difference?" Dave felt that "if the first doctor had been more forthright and told us what he was looking for and why, we might have sought out a second opinion, maybe gone to an oncologist and had a little different agenda." Like these three, many people believe, and with some justification, that if their cancer had been properly diagnosed with the first symptoms, their chances of survival could have been greater. So when the diagnosis is finally confirmed, this anger at the medical people is normal and is the result of built-up frustration. Although anger is generally considered a self-defeating emotion, when dealing with cancer, some anger can be viewed as healthy. It indicates a person's active involvement in life.

Denial

Confronting the diagnosis with denial is also healthy, to a point. Initially, denial makes it possible to go about life's normal routines during the early period of adjustment. Since absorbing a cancer diagnosis takes time, without some denial, a person could be paralyzed and unable to function for days. Also, denial gives you time to start building a bridge of hope. That sense of hope is a key factor that sustains people and helps them continue normal participation in social and work-related activities.

Denial benefits the patient early in the illness, but long-term denial can distort reality and impede the proper course of treatment. People with cancer and their families should watch for signs that indicate denial is being used to avoid confronting the facts of the illness. In most cases, early diagnosis and prompt treatment are critical to success. If a person's unhealthy denial seems to be delaying treatment, family members might ask when the next scheduled doctor's appointment will be and suggest going along. Or they could decide as a family to attend a support group or educational course like I CAN COPE. If family members act in a way that is open and not fearful, the person with cancer can accept the diagnosis more easily. Getting beyond denial is necessary before the family can begin to work effectively with the treatment team.

Sadness and Depression

Depression has been defined as anger turned inward. If anger cannot be openly expressed, once denial is finally replaced with reality, depression commonly occurs. For people with cancer, depression is usually the result of feeling helpless. One day you are strong and vital and in control of your life. The next day you find out you have cancer. The control is lost. People begin to feel that the cancer, the medical team, and their family members are controlling their lives. When people see their health fading and they no longer feel in control of their own destiny, they begin to question their self-worth. Almost overnight, this active, productive family member has become a dependent invalid. Malinda described it well when she said, "All the things I used to think were nothing now had become a big deal. Getting out of bed to go to the bathroom made me faint. Eating a little piece of candy made me vomit."

Dave's depression and loss of control actually occurred before his diagnosis. He knew something was wrong; he was having severe chills, fevers, and body aches. Yet no one seemed able to identify the ailment. Dave remembers the anxiety, uncertainty, and lack of control from those circumstances as being the worst months of the whole cancer experience. And the cancer hadn't even been identified yet.

Helping Someone Who is Depressed

Depression is a normal, appropriate response to a cancer diagnosis. But family and friends may be uncomfortable witnessing it. No one enjoys seeing a loved one grieving or downcast, so we attempt to cheer them up. Yet, family and friends must remember that no one can bring another person out of a depression.

The best strategy for helping a depressed person is to offer a safe, supportive environment. The following guidelines may also be of assistance:

- Allow your loved one the temporary luxury of self-pity when there are obvious reasons for being depressed. People work through depression most effectively by expressing feelings. Sitting quietly while a depressed person cries, or offering a gentle touch, speaks louder and more effectively than words.

- Avoid worn-out cliches such as "Everything will be all right," or "Don't worry, things will work out." False words of encouragement do more harm than good and are more destructive than saying nothing at all. Instead, carefully assess the circumstances and focus on the realistic, hopeful signs you honestly believe exist.

- Be supportive, but don't try to control a depressed person's feelings. Any attempt by family or friends to exert control may simply lengthen the depression. People must work through their own depression. For people with cancer, control is all important. Their downcast mood may miraculously change when they start to feel in control again. Being involved in the treatment process sometimes diminishes feelings of helplessness.

Helping Yourself Through Depression

If you are depressed, remember that overcoming depression takes time and effort. The following strategies may help you work through your depression:

- Acknowledge that some things are out of your control.

- Consider what options are available to you now.

- Develop a master plan allowing you to use the options you choose.

- Take a small, first step toward putting your plan into action.

Sadness and depression about the disease and its treatment are normal. But sometimes that depression is more serious and starts feeling worse than simply being sad. People can become depressed about themselves rather than the illness. This type of depression is more long term. They may lose all interest in things that used to give them pleasure, sleep too much or too little, lose their appetite, feel constantly tired, lose their ability to think clearly or concentrate, and harbor feelings of worthlessness or excessive guilt. These symptoms aren't short term and may last six weeks to two months. This kind of depression should be handled by a professional. Psychotherapy may work for some, antidepressant medication for others, or sometimes a combination of the two is most effective. Family members should be watchful and make sure a depressed person gets medical help as quickly as possible.

Uncertainty

To accept cancer means to accept uncertainty in your life. One participant in an I CAN COPE class explained it well when he said: "When we are born, we are given a pack of cards for life, face down. As life unfolds, the cards come up and must be played. When my cancer came up, I had to play it. What was my alternative? My choice was not if to play it, but how to play it."

People with cancer must learn to erase the word "cure" from their vocabulary. "I'm healthy, I don't have any signs of cancer right now, but I can't say I'm cured," Bill comments. After 10 years in remission, Bill finally had to acknowledge that cancer, like heart disease and diabetes, is a chronic illness. Contrary to the popular myth that "cancer is something you die from," cancer should be viewed as something "you can learn to live with."

Even when treatment is completed and all symptoms are gone, people still live with the possibility that the cancer may recur. The anxiety is always present. One person referred to it as sitting on top of a time bomb. Plans for future vacations, new homes, and especially retirement all become more tenuous when the thought of cancer's recurrence remains uppermost in people's minds.

Dave refused to give in to such feelings, even though he acknowledges that recurrence is a possibility. And he hopes that Loretta isn't dwelling on that uncertainty either. "I'd like her to feel there is no uncertainty, that we can still live a normal life." Yet Loretta seems puzzled by Dave's reaction. Unlike many cancer survivors, Dave isn't anxious to make any major changes in his life. "Don't change anything. That's Dave," Loretta comments. "I've never heard Dave say, 'All my life I've wanted to do this or that, and now I'm going to do it.'" But Dave's pragmatic nature and genuine love for Loretta both come through when he responds: "Where's the icing on the cake? It's already there. We've had a rich full life." For Dave, life today is as good as it gets, so the uncertainty about tomorrow doesn't cloud his vision.

Experienced cancer "veterans" suggest the following as techniques for learning to live with uncertainty.

- *Give up the role of a sick person and get on with living.* Most people want to resume their previous role as soon as possible and show the world they are well. Family members can help by adopting an attitude of wellness in the household.

- *Begin to focus on the quality, not the quantity, of life.* People who have been through the cancer experience are livers of life. They offer tremendous insight into what is really important. Lou often says, "It's surprising, but it took the cancer for me to realize there is so much more to life than having a clean house." Lothair is philosophical about the uncertainty. He says, "It's the human condition—life and death. I just know a little bit more about my ending than other people. Probably." People who learn to adapt and live one day at a time are victorious regardless of how long they live.

- *Focus on what you have, not on what you have lost.* Helping others, especially newly diagnosed cancer patients, seems to help many people cope with the uncertainty. Cansurmount and Reach to Recovery, both sponsored by the American Cancer Society, are two programs that depend on volunteers to work one-on-one with newly diagnosed cancer patients.

One of Malinda's first hospital visitors was a young Reach to Recovery volunteer who had the same breast surgery the previous year. After hearing her story and seeing how healthy she was, Malinda felt hopeful about her own recovery.

Fear

What we do not know, we cannot possess. And there is much we do not know about cancer. Did they get it all? Will I have further treatment? Will it be painful? Will it recur? How long will I live? Most people will never know the answer to all these questions. And when cancer is first diagnosed, the fear caused by these unknowns produces more anxiety than the fear of pain or death. As knowledge is accumulated, fear subsides. In addition to fear of the unknown, four other distinct fears are also reported—fear of alienation, fear of mutilation, fear of death, and fear of losing control.

Fear of Alienation

People with cancer often call themselves "the new lepers." A spouse suddenly loses interest in sex. Friends stop calling. Grown children become distant and patronizing. People with cancer feel abandoned and isolated. They are no longer acceptable as lover, parent, or friend.

Well-meaning friends and relatives often fuel this fear, usually reacting because of their attitude about the disease, not about the person. Loved ones are afraid of cancer. Some still believe it is contagious. Many are convinced their loved one is going to die and they withdraw emotionally in preparation for that death. Alienation is common and can lead to depression or despair. Family and friends can help.

- Ask other friends and relatives to call or visit regularly.

- Suggest a cancer support group or attend one yourself.

- Seek advice from social workers, nurses, or clergy.

Fear of Mutilation

When treatment involves surgery, fear of mutilation almost always occurs. Losing the affected body part represents many losses—of belonging, of self-worth, of life as it used to be. Feeling no longer whole, people with cancer often retreat from normal activities and exhibit the classic symptoms of depression. They suffer from insomnia and loss of appetite and have difficulty concentrating.

Being wheeled into an operating room is a time of great vulnerability. Not only are people afraid of surgery and its possible disfigurement, but their sexuality is also threatened. Some people fear surgery so much that they reject potentially curative surgery.

Fear of Death

More than anything, cancer brings a person face to face with death. Even when the prognosis is good, death is more real than it was before the cancer diagnosis. Although it may not be fatal, cancer is life threatening. And because death is a possible outcome, it too must be faced.

Many find great strength in religion as they wrestle with their own mortality. Being able to rely on a greater power for courage and hope is sometimes the key to coping successfully with the possibility of death.

Fear of a lingering, painful death is mentioned more often than fear of death itself. As discussed in Chapter 3, great strides have been made in the field of pain control in the last several years. Most people are able to get relief from pain if they are willing to be assertive and make their wishes known.

Fear of Losing Control

Fear of becoming dependent and helpless is most intense in people who place a high value on independence. Cancer is a controlling force. The disease controls the body. The medical team controls the treatment. What is left for the patient to control?

People who are particularly threatened are those whose self-esteem lies in taking care of or supporting others. If breadwinners cannot work or homemakers cannot perform their normal duties, they feel they have lost control of their environment. Friends and loved ones can minimize this fear by doing the following:

- Treat the person with cancer as a capable, responsible person.

- Make sure your need to help isn't at the expense of the other person's independence.

- Emphasize the things within a person's control, such as diet, relationships with friends, exercise, relaxation techniques, spirituality, and goal setting.

- Help the person stay involved in family decision making and in decisions affecting medical treatment.

James Baldwin said, "Not everything that is faced can be changed. But nothing can be changed until it is faced." Facing cancer head-on is frightening. If you are the person with cancer, surely you have experienced many of these new conditions. Find it reassuring to know that you are not alone.

Communicating Feelings

While going through the turmoil of everything cancer involves, you naturally expect to receive much-needed support and understanding from those closest to you—spouse, parents, or children. You are certain you will be able to rely on family and friends to buoy you up. After all, you're the one who has the cancer.

But remember that those closest to you are riding the same roller coaster. They are experiencing the same kinds of feelings, and at the same time. If you are shocked, so are they. If you are angry, they might be even more angry. And when two people are angry or afraid or feeling helpless, their ability to communicate is severely inhibited. Don't be surprised if family and friends are unable to offer support in the beginning. But once the shock has passed, everyone should be able to recognize that feelings are manageable. The notion that feelings rule people's lives and render them helpless is simply not true. But gaining control over your feelings means learning how to share them with others.

Fear Inhibits Communication

Debbie had never really established a close relationship with her father, so his aloofness when learning of her cancer was not surprising. But at a time like this, she expected more. Whenever Debbie's cancer was mentioned, he would simply get a pained look on his face. "When I told him about the diagnosis, he said about two words and walked out the front door," she remembers. "That was the last I saw of him that night. I know he was hurting, but why couldn't he let anybody see that?" Yet later, she knew he was thinking of her. When her parents went grocery shopping, her dad took a second cart through the store to "do some shopping for Debbie." He didn't know what to say to her, but he felt a need to do something.

When both the person with cancer and the close family member are afraid, that fear often gets in the way of the very thing they need most. What Debbie wanted and needed was for her father to say what he was feeling, to tell her his fears so she could in turn share hers. But he couldn't. What did they both fear? The word "cancer" is enough to frighten most of us. In general, people know very little about cancer, and fear of the unknown creates anxiety.

Several studies have shown that both physical contact (hand holding, etc.) and talking help dissipate fear and panic. If Debbie's father had put his arm around her and, through his body language, given her permission to talk about what had happened, both of them probably would have felt better.

Gathering information about cancer and its treatment reduces anxiety for many people. Most want to discuss their cancer right away and usually end up talking to doctors, nurses, or other cancer patients. When people have the opportunity to touch and hold one another in addition to talking, they gain strength from the combination of knowledge and physical contact. If people are able to begin forming a positive attitude about their illness, it becomes easier to cultivate the will to live and the desire to fight.

Stay Close, Listen, and Accept

Debbie ended up getting most of her support from people who made it comfortable for her to openly express how she felt. "The people who helped me the most were not the ones who denied what I was feeling. Instead of saying 'Oh, don't worry about it,' they let me tell them exactly what I was going through without getting freaked out by it. When people first learn they have cancer, they need someone who will let them be themselves. My advice to family and friends who don't know what to say or do would be to stay close. Check in regularly to see how they are doing. It's a way of showing you care. Be available, but don't bug them."

Research has shown that people who choose to openly express their thoughts and feelings about their cancer adapt more easily than those who don't. Getting thoughts out in the open not only affords people the opportunity to get in touch with their own feelings, but is also an excellent way of providing emotional catharsis.

Emotional Reactions Vary

After Jim's surgery, he and Shirley were told there was no further treatment recommended for his leiomyosarcoma. Since Jim's cancer was rare and involved the muscle lining of his stomach, the only treatment recommended at the time was removal of the tumor. There was no indication the cancer had spread, so follow-up chemotherapy was not suggested. "Knowing nothing about cancer or its treatment at the time, we believed them," Jim remembers. He decided to take an early retirement soon after that, and during the next year he and Shirley traveled around the country and rarely spoke of his cancer. He says, "I was feeling good at the time. We were both convinced we had conquered it."

Fear set in the following year when Jim again started feeling run down. "Even before I went in to see the doctor, I knew the cancer was back." Tests revealed abnormal liver function. The cancer had returned and was now in Jim's liver.

"When the doctor told me it had settled in his liver, I panicked," Shirley admits. "I knew enough about cancer to know that when it gets to the liver, it's bad." Her fear threw her into high gear. She went on the offense, making her own plans and mapping out strategies for attacking what she now referred to as "our cancer." But the news evoked a totally different response from Jim.

Jim's reaction was one of despair. With the cancer's return, he saw his independence fading. He immediately began painting the house, despite his weakness. He wondered who would finish the painting? Who would do all the chores he had always done? Jim saw himself becoming a burden to his family. He felt guilty about Shirley devoting all her time and energy to his care at the expense of her own interests.

People with cancer often add extra baggage to their burden by feeling responsible for the distress of others. "I'm such a burden to my family" is a statement often heard and aptly describes Jim's guilty feelings. Instead of feeling responsible for their spouse, parent, or child, people with cancer need to concentrate on taking care of their own needs. Although it is wise to be open and willing to accept the family's involvement and interest, it is unwise to accept the responsibility for how they are feeling.

Depression is Normal

As Shirley busied herself with a new nutrition program, organizing support systems, and setting up a prayer chain, she repressed any negative emotions. She refused to cry. "Tears came to my eyes," she says, "but in two years, I haven't cried yet. The day will come, but I don't have time right now." Her insistence on showing outward strength may have made it hard for Jim to recognize and work through his own despair. With Shirley holding back, he may have found it difficult to openly express his own grief.

Mood swings and depression are normal. Loved ones can help by standing by and not denying negative feelings. Shirley needed to understand that in addition to being strong, she also needed to be receptive to whatever Jim was feeling. They both learned through experience that sharing negative thoughts is normal and necessary, even though listening to them is sometimes painful. Shirley summed it up when she said, "I finally realized there were many things I couldn't do for Jim, including taking away his depression. But I could listen."

Listen Without Judging

When you let the person with cancer know you are willing to listen, you are telling them three things:

- It is all right to talk and express feelings to me.

- You can share your problems and concerns with me.

- You are important and I care about you.

Communication is never a one-way street. Jim and Shirley were both going through dramatic emotional changes, but their feelings were actually quite different. They needed to get their differences out in the open. When they were honest about their emotions, both ended up feeling less isolated and fearful.

Love and Support

Bill had always had a loving relationship with both his parents. And although, like Debbie, he was young and unmarried, he found it much easier to discuss his cancer with his family. In fact, Bill says he doesn't remember a time that his parents weren't around when he needed them. And that included when the cancer was diagnosed. "They were at the World's Fair," he recalls. "I ruined their vacation by calling to tell them about the surgery. They came home immediately."

Bill's mother, a registered nurse, was extremely supportive. She also helped him understand the various details of his cancer and the medical procedures he would be going through. "That helped me immensely. Just having somebody who knew what was happening."

Bill's dad had always preached to him that "knowledge is power." His parents encouraged him to learn all he could about his cancer and suggested the I CAN COPE classes. They were available to listen when he wanted to talk. Although he owned his own house, his parents brought him home to live with them while he was recuperating from surgery and during his drug treatment. "My parents really did everything possible for me. They even bought me a new water bed because I wasn't sleeping well. They thought maybe if I had a new bed, I would sleep better. My dad is a real positive thinker. He truly believes in the power of positive thinking. I think that had a real effect on how I went through all this."

Bill believes his successful recovery was due in part to the fact that his negative emotions didn't grow all out of proportion. His fears were held in check by knowledge of his disease. Depression was minimized because his close relationships remained positive and supportive. He was able to focus all his emotional energy on supporting his medical team to help him get well.

Ten years later, when Bill's cancer recurred, Bill responded in much the same way. Married now and living in a new home, he once again received love and support from family and refused to let negative thoughts get in the way of his recovery. "The new antinausea medication made it easier to stay positive this time, because I felt so much better," Bill says. "To keep out negative thoughts, I encourage people to stay busy. Find something you enjoy doing, then do it." Looking around Bill's home, you can see he has surrounded himself with things he enjoys—his lawn tractor, a trampoline, bikes, a camper, and an assortment of cars and trucks he can tinker with. "Sometimes the body breaks down, just like a car," he muses. "You fix it and then you get on with your life."

Testing the Strength of a Marriage

Ideally, people with cancer should keep their emotions as stable as possible. "But how do you keep your emotions stable when you feel your whole life is falling apart?" Malinda posed that question shortly after her husband announced he was taking a new job in another state while she was still receiving drug treatment in Minneapolis. "My husband took it very hard, and still does. He's just not facing up to the reality of it all." She admits they were already experiencing some marital problems anyway. But Malinda believes the cancer could have pulled them together. Instead, it tested their marriage to the breaking point.

Yet Malinda is philosophical as she explores the reasons why the cancer pushed them apart instead of pulling them together. She believes a spouse needs to be totally involved, as painful as that may be, in every aspect of the cancer patient's treatment. But it is clear that her husband was not. "He wasn't there after the surgery when the doctor gave me the bad news. Later on, when the doctor explained about the chemotherapy, he wasn't there either. I keep thinking that maybe if he had been there to hear first hand about some of that, he would be better at coping now." During the difficult early times in the hospital, Malinda needed someone by her side for support. The first night after surgery is often the most painful—emotionally and physically. Having someone close by at all times provides reassurance. "If that person had been him, if he had been forced to help at the hardest time, he would understand me better now."

But Malinda endured the hardest times alone. And as her husband retreated both physically and emotionally, the chasm between them widened. "The hardest time is when you have hit rock bottom. That is when you really need someone with you. Someone to grow with you. Someone who has seen you through the low point and who is able to understand you as you move up the ladder toward acceptance." In this young marriage, a strong enough bond had not been forged to allow for that kind of growth.

Dave was fortunate to have someone with him all the way through his cancer journey. For him, rock bottom seemed to have occurred before the diagnosis, when his symptoms were most profound. "I was getting no sleep and constantly wondering what was wrong with me. I even kept a journal of my symptoms." But Loretta was tuned in every step of the way. The surgeon who finally diagnosed Dave's cancer was actually a colleague of Loretta's. She had worked with him in the hospital, knew of his expertise, and trusted him implicitly.

When Dave's cancer recurred and he realized the bone marrow transplant was his only real chance for success, his hospitalization became a shared experience. "Loretta planned to be with me every evening, bring a change of clothes for me, and eat with me. These things kept a sense of normalcy in our lives." Dave and Loretta worked together as a team to find normalcy in a life that had been disrupted by cancer. They both accepted the seriousness of the condition, then tried to maintain a forward-looking attitude. "We had our low points," Dave admits, "and our high points. And we had a lot of laughs."

"Laughter very close to tears sometimes," Loretta interjects.

This marriage was tested by cancer and grew. Dave and Loretta seemed to achieve what was so elusive to Malinda and her husband—having someone to grow with you up the ladder of acceptance.

Malinda's husband was never able to accept the seriousness of her condition. When she broached the topic, he'd throw up his hands and say, "Do we have to talk about this again?" Still, Malinda learned some valuable lessons from the experience. "I suppose it would have been easier with him holding my hand. But the good side of my story is that I have had to muster the courage within myself because I didn't have him to lean on. I had to do it on my own." By denying the seriousness of her condition, he communicated a lack of interest. By not being with her, he communicated a lack of sincerity.

To the contrary, Loretta understood and acknowledged the seriousness of Dave's condition. And she showed her sincerity and commitment in a multitude of ways. "She drove herself to do it all," Dave says. "She was working full time, maintaining the household, keeping up correspondence with friends about my condition, and yet was my constant support." Dave's hospital journal notes only one evening spent without Loretta by his side.

The Value of Friends

Malinda knew she needed support, so she turned to her parents and friends. Her reaching out to others yielded a tremendous response. "I didn't know I had such good friends until now." Through friends, she made contact with a recently widowed female artist who invited Malinda to move in with her. "Evie has taken me in and treats me like a daughter. She knows all about me and isn't afraid to talk about my cancer. She is always available to listen without judging me." Evie's large home in a quiet neighborhood near a lake afforded Malinda plenty of space of her own.

Other friends helped Malinda get back to normal by taking her shopping and including her in their day-to-day activities. "A friend had a lingerie party and asked me to come. I felt so embarrassed. Everybody was in the bedroom trying things on. I didn't want to take my clothes off. But everyone acted so normal. At the time, I was still very self-conscious. Now, when I look back, I realize how good it was for me. They were brave to invite me, then just act like everything was normal." Someone with cancer doesn't want to talk about it all the time. Sometimes they just want to forget their cancer and go about life as if everything is normal.

Asking for Help

For Malinda, who was young and very active, adjusting to dependency was a problem. "It was real humiliating for someone who was perfectly healthy, who was running and swimming two days earlier, to now be dependent on others. It was a very hard time."

Who wants to be a burden to others? No one! When you have always been healthy and are used to helping others, adjusting to being the recipient of help is a difficult transition to make. But the person with cancer often needs help. And that means learning to ask. Malinda remembers a time in particular when she had to do just that.

She says, "Once I had to take a taxi to the hospital for my treatment because my husband couldn't get off work to take me. That was before I learned to be brave enough to ask friends for help. That was a big breakthrough for me. Learning to say, 'Would you help me?' It's so hard when you've never had to do it before." Usually, friends and loved ones want to help, but they just don't know what to do and are waiting to be asked.

Malinda learned to ask, and the response she received was overwhelming. "Just the fact that I would ask seemed to make my friends feel better." Most people feel helpless. Being able to do something for a friend makes them feel more supportive. "Seeing the generosity of those people provided me with a whole new definition of friendship."

The Changing Face of Friendships

Like Malinda, most people with cancer will tell you this experience teaches you who your true friends are. Jim was also quick to point that out. He says, "We've lost some friends since this happened to me. But we have also seen how important our really good friends are. Some of our strongest friendships have developed with people we have met since I learned about my cancer." When asked why he thought he and his wife lost friends, he replied, "Some people just can't handle talking about this, or watching me go through it. I can understand that, and I appreciate their honesty. I would probably be the same way."

Sometimes the changing face of friendships involves cultivating new friendships. Debbie and Malinda found a true kinship after first meeting at an I CAN COPE class. Similar in age and disposition, the two young women could truly understand and empathize with one another and could communicate on a higher level because of the similarity of their experiences. "I think it's much different when you're 28 than when you're 58," they both agree. Finding one another was fortunate. Lou and Ingvar met John and Hazel at I CAN COPE classes, too. Again, the similar nature of their circumstances created a fertile environment for a budding friendship. Similar in age, they shared common concerns, both as individuals and as couples. "After class, we often had a bite to eat together," John remembers. All four people could talk comfortably, knowing that cancer can be a natural part of the conversation.

Jim noticed that old social patterns changed. "When you're not healthy, it's hard to go with other people who are healthy. In a way, it changes your social structure. For awhile, I was going out for lunch with the guys I used to work with. Everyone else looked really healthy. I knew I didn't look that good. That's hard to cope with—for them and for me. You want to be the same as before, but you aren't. Things have changed."

That change needn't be bad. Using cancer as a motivation for change often improves quality of life. Letting go of people, things, or jobs that are not supportive of a person's physical or emotional well being should be seen as a positive step. Through a process of reevaluation, you can perhaps free yourself from unhealthy relationships or situations.

Good friends will be sensitive enough to realize that life has changed for the person with cancer. They will take the time to ask about it and will truly want to listen.

Talking About Your Cancer

Lou remembers that after her cancer diagnosis, her feelings of isolation were magnified by the silence of her friends. "So many people are uptight, especially outsiders," she says. "Many of my friends stopped calling me after they found out. So I got on the phone and called them. I talked very openly about it. From then on, we got along fine. I really believe if you have cancer, you've got to be the first to talk about it. That gives your friends permission to be open with you." Lou calls herself a "blabbermouth." "I blabber about this disease as if it were no more serious than a sliver in my finger." But her willingness to be open with others instantly makes them feel comfortable.

Dave discovered that people were anxious to learn about the details of having a bone marrow transplant. Many had heard the term but were unfamiliar with its meaning. "Even doctor friends would ask about exactly what happens," Dave says. "They know the medical terminology, but I think it's interesting for them to hear the layman's actual experience of going through it." Dave helped himself and others by talking about the transplant. Telling the story seemed to be therapeutic for him. And Dave's positive experience demystified the whole process. After listening to him tell the story, bone marrow transplant sounds far less frightening.

Personal Experience Aids Communication

Talking about cancer can be difficult. Because friends don't know what to say and are afraid of hurting feelings, they often choose to say nothing. Finding a friend or relative who has had some personal experience with cancer may make the initial conversation easier. Lou recalls helping a friend open up after learning of her own cancer. "After finding out," Lou says, "she couldn't talk about it at all. She couldn't even say the word, 'cancer.'" Lou and Ingvar invited the friend and her husband to dinner. "At dinner, I started jabbering about myself. I was feeling good, Ingvar says I was looking good, and I was happy. I was sympathetic with her, because I had been there. I told her I knew how she felt. And I did. I've been through it myself." At that point, the friend opened up and started to discuss her illness. She admitted how hard it had been to share her feelings with anyone. They ended up having a good discussion in which even her husband became comfortable enough to expose his own fears.

Initiating Discussion of Uncomfortable Thoughts and Feelings

The Patient Might Say:

• I feel like my cancer has made us strangers, and I'm becoming isolated and alienated from you. Right now we're suffering privately. Is there anything I can do to help you through this time? We've been dancing around this issue a lot lately. Can't we find a way to really talk?

• It's hard for me to even say the word cancer, much less tell you my feelings about my illness. And I'm afraid it will upset you if I bring it up.

The Family Member or Friends Might Say:

• Some things are hard to think about, much less talk about. But if you ever want to talk, I'm more than willing to listen.

• You seem quite calm about all of this, so I've tried not to get you upset with my feelings. But your cancer has me frightened.

• I wish it were easier for us to talk about all the pain you have been through. But I'm afraid if we start talking I'd break down and cry, and you wouldn't like that.

• It doesn't help when you tell me not to worry. I am worried. It upsets me when you make jokes and tell me there is nothing to worry about.

Adapted from *The Road Back to Health* by Neil A. Fiore, Ph.D.

Communicating With Your Doctor

Throughout history, doctors have been revered, eventually becoming one of the most powerful professional groups in America. Most people grew up believing doctor's decisions were always right and tended to put "the good doctor" on a pedestal. Do what the doctor orders, don't question the decision, and be polite.

But as more and more people are becoming interested in the mind-body connection and increasingly wary of all the high-tech, expensive medicine, we are beginning to see a change in that perception. People are now acknowledging that the doctor-patient relationship needs to be a two-way street. They are starting to question their doctors and to seek second opinions before undertaking any major medical procedures. People with cancer are particularly encouraged to seek second opinions if they are questioning a doctor's prognosis.

Most doctors want to talk to you, but maybe not as much as you want to talk. In fact, doctors spend an average of 1.3 minutes giving information, and patients spend an average of 8 seconds asking questions during a normal 16-minute office visit. For this reason, it is important that you plan your doctor visits carefully to ensure maximum communication. Both the doctor and the patient must contribute if their communication is to be successful.

Keeping up Your End of the Conversation

Because every cancer is unique, providing detailed information about your condition is vital. Often, just the fact that you are feeling better is one clue a doctor uses to assess how well your treatment is working, and vice versa.

This was true in Jim's case. After his recurrence, the doctors put him back on chemotherapy. Without good reporting from Jim, it would be hard for the doctor to assess how well Jim's body was tolerating the drug. After completing treatment, Jim reported he was feeling better, had more energy, and his appetite had returned. "I told the doctor that I really felt good," Jim says. Jim's report led the doctor to believe that his cancer was currently being controlled.

The Importance of Giving Complete Information

People who are in tune with their bodies and who report thoroughly make it easier for the doctor to accurately assess the success of a treatment program. Any changes in body function should be reported, even if they seem unimportant. Never withhold information out of fear or because you think it might not be significant.

Lou, who was always tuned in to her body, was cancer free for many years. She was hospitalized twice for pain, and although she had numerous tests, they revealed nothing. "All along, I kept telling the doctors I thought it was the cancer returning. The pain was located in the area of my liver. At the time, they said, 'No, not after all these years.' I wasn't convinced, so I found a different doctor." Finally the new doctor confirmed that Lou's cancer had recurred in her liver, just as she had suspected. Lou was aware of her body and how it was changing. She understood the importance of communicating those changes to her doctor as clearly and completely as possible.

Getting the Most from Your Appointments

Start with a list that includes questions you want to ask as well as information you want to tell the doctor. Start the list the day you make your appointment and keep it tacked up in an obvious place where you can add to it easily. Encourage family members to add their questions.

During your appointment, take notes on the doctor's answers for review at home. If you think you won't remember everything, take along a tape recorder and record your visit. That way, family or friends can hear the information first hand. Most of the time, people like to have a family member or friend along during discussions with the doctor. That way, you have someone with whom you can discuss the answers. Also, another person is often able to clarify something you didn't understand, or may have a different interpretation of what was said.

Family conferences are also available when decisions must be made regarding treatment options. A family conference allows the entire family an opportunity to be together with the doctors in order to avoid misunderstandings.

Insist on the Best—For You

The doctor-patient relationship is sacred when dealing with a chronic, life-threatening disease. Do you believe your relationship is one of real trust and confidence? Do you come away from a visit feeling the doctor has taken the time to really listen to you? Even if you did not hear exactly what you wanted to, do you feel you and your doctor are working together as a team? Do you sense a bond is being formed between you and your doctor? If you are unable to answer those questions with a yes or if you believe you and your doctor are just not on the same wavelength, now may be the time to consider a new doctor. Continue looking until you find someone with whom you are comfortable, someone you can work with on a partnership basis and someone in whom you have utmost confidence.

Malinda liked her first doctor immediately, "I appreciated his honesty and his straight-forward, punching style. That's why I stuck with him all along. I want someone to tell me the truth, no matter how brutal. I don't want someone to beat around the bush." Other people may be very uncomfortable with that style, and they would be better off looking for a doctor with a more subtle, less direct approach. Malinda's doctor had a style that fit her personality and she stayed with him until his practice moved East. By that time, she knew what she was looking for in a doctor.

The oncologist who was recommended to her was part of a large, well-known practice, and Malinda anticipated she would be treated well. She was not particularly impressed on her first visit, but chose to go back for a second appointment. "I was having an ache in my back that was not going away. I asked for a bone scan. He said to me, 'Every time you have an ache or pain, you can't be thinking you have cancer.' I told him, 'I've had this before, and I think I should know what it feels like.' He said if it would make me happy, he would order a bone scan. Can you believe it? Make me happy."

After that appointment, Malinda began the search for a new doctor. She even went so far as to call a doctor at M.D. Anderson Cancer Hospital in Houston to ask for advice. Based on the recommendation of the Houston doctor, Malinda contacted an oncologist in Minneapolis and saw him the next day. "I liked him immediately. He sat right down, took the files, and we went through them page by page, discussing everything. We were together over two hours." During that time, the doctor telephoned for the results of Malinda's bone scan. "He came back with bad news. The cancer had recurred in the lumbar region of the spine."

Malinda's news was not encouraging. But she was encouraged that she found a doctor who respected her wishes and would work with her. "He even asked if it was okay to call Houston to discuss my case. I was delighted he was doing that."

Treatment—It's Your Choice

Although the doctor recommends potential treatment strategies, the patient is ultimately responsible for saying yes or no to that program. If you feel uncomfortable with the path a doctor has chosen, you should speak up—and be prepared to say why. If a discussion doesn't convince you, seek a second opinion.

Lou ran into just such a situation when it was discovered that her cancer had recurred in the liver. When tests finally confirmed the cancer, her doctor said treatment must begin immediately.

"He scared the living daylights out of me," Lou admits. "He was so intense. I was certain I could die anytime." The doctor convinced her that the best route was to go with a conventional chemotherapy program for one year. She would be in the hospital for three days every three weeks. "It was a miserable year. By year's end, I was feeling sick from one treatment right on into the next," Lou remembers.

When Lou saw her doctor to discuss the next step, she was disappointed in his suggestion. She says, "He advised having another year of chemo. I said, 'You're crazy. I'd rather die.' " Lou was at a point where her decision differed from her doctor's decision. She chose her present quality of life over what she envisioned life would be like if she continued with another year of chemotherapy. Her doctor accepted her decision and offered surgery as an alternative.

Lou's oncologist referred her to the Mayo Clinic. She saw three surgeons before finding one with expertise in cancer surgery, particularly of the liver. "He told me he could take the tumor out of my liver. And, because it was a slow-growing cancer, he thought I would be okay for quite a while."

Lou's surgery was successful, and it bought her two more comfortable years before she began having other symptoms. By speaking up when her doctor suggested another year of chemotherapy, Lou was able to find a more acceptable form of treatment. She was also fortunate that her doctor respected her wishes and decision. His willingness to make the necessary appointments at Mayo Clinic was a sign that he really cared about his patient.

Finding the Right Chemistry

Perhaps it seems silly to talk about personal chemistry when dealing with a serious subject like cancer. But each doctor-patient relationship is unique. How well it works is influenced by a variety of factors, including your personality, the doctor's personality, your age, your sex, your type of cancer, and the doctor's philosophy about treating it. Just because a friend or family member recommends a doctor doesn't necessarily mean he or she is the right one for you.

Malinda went to a popular Minnesota clinic for a second opinion when her cancer first metastasized. She was both surprised and disappointed at how the initial visit went. "The doctor told me to expect a miracle. So I got mad at him and said, 'I resent the fact that you want to talk about miracles and I want to talk about treatment.' The doctor just sat there with his feet up on the desk, leaning back in his chair and rocking. I felt he was being patronizing and told him so."

This same doctor might have responded differently to another person under different circumstances. For whatever reason, he was unable to deal with Malinda in a manner that made her feel confident about his care.

When you choose a doctor, you are in the driver's seat. It is your health—and your pocketbook—that are involved. If you want to play an active role in your treatment program, make that very clear at the outset. If your doctor is less than enthusiastic about that kind of relationship, you have the choice to keep looking until you are satisfied. But be certain your decision is based on reality and not on a desire to find a doctor who promises an easy fix or treatment free of pain or anxiety. When you find the right doctor, you'll know. Then go through the list at the end of this chapter, "Are We Communicating? Ten Steps to a Terrific Doctor-Patient Relationship," and use it to help you cultivate a good relationship with the doctor you have chosen.

Taking Time to Communicate

A radiation oncologist, talking about the doctor-patient relationship, gave this advice. "I think one of the most important things a patient can do is simply try to be very straightforward. When wanting to know about a certain problem related to cancer, be very open in asking what is happening. When patients are sincere, when they identify what they want to know and why, most doctors will recognize that sincerity and will take the time to develop the relationship."

"Unfortunately, I think often doctors are guilty of getting busy and running back and forth to different hospitals and getting involved in too many things. We end up not having the time to spend with patients that we should."

"There is always room for improvement in doctor-patient communication. Where we doctors often fall down is in not talking to our patients enough; that is one of the most frequent complaints I hear. Sometimes we think we know a little bit too much, or we aren't as sincere as we should be. When we're dealing with cancer, one of the first things we all need is humility. None of us has the perfect answer."

Doctors may occasionally need to be reminded there are no easy answers when dealing with cancer. People with cancer may need to learn to be more assertive and ask for what they need. If you feel your doctor is spending too little time with you, ask to have more time scheduled for your next appointment. Come prepared with the specific items you wish to discuss. Being straightforward about your questions and concerns makes it easier for the doctor to give appropriate responses.

If you believe your doctor has not answered any of these questions completely, ask more questions. To the greatest degree possible, you need to know what to expect in the months and years ahead, so be persistent.

Questions to Ask Your Doctor

- What type of cancer do I have, and what is the medical name?

- Has the cancer spread beyond the original site? To where?

- Will I need more tests after this? What will they be?

- What treatment do you recommend? Why?

- What are the risks and benefits of this treatment?

- Are other treatment options available?

Doctors, patients, loved ones, and friends all share in the responsibility of learning to understand the emotions surrounding a cancer diagnosis. The family's mobile, which once was spinning around wildly, eventually does come to rest. Acceptance slowly begins to replace the chaotic, high-strung emotions most people feel upon first learning of their cancer. When all parties involved deal with these emotions openly and honestly, the result should be a healthy acceptance of this lifestyle change. The following pages provide insight into specific types of language that either enhance or inhibit communication.

Communication Enhancers

Concerned Silence. This is probably the most difficult technique to carry out. Many people are uncomfortable with silence and feel that someone should always be talking. Silence is golden, especially when important information is being shared. Allow time for silence, along with supportive actions such as intermittent eye contact, leaning forward, and handholding.

Encouragement. Often people need verbal permission to share thoughts and feelings. Statements like, "I'd like to hear more about that," and "If you would like to share that with me, I'd be glad to listen," show interest and willingness to become involved in the conversation. This technique can also be useful if the conversation is bogged down.

Prompters. This technique lets the sender know that you are still listening, that you understand, accept, and empathize. Short phrases such as "I see," "Yes," and "Aha" often will encourage additional conversation without interrupting the sender's train of thought.

Restatement. To help you understand thoughts and feelings, it is often useful to feed back what you have heard or thought you have heard. The sender says, "I am so sick and tired of being in the hospital." You can say, "You are tired of being hospitalized." This helps the sender understand the impressions conveyed by specific choices of words and helps to clarify feelings.

Reflection. Put the factual portion of the sender's statement in your own words and send it back for clarification. The sender says, "I'm afraid I'll never be well again." Say, "That's a real concern for you now." This technique helps to clarify your understanding of the message and allows the sender an opportunity to correct your statement if your assessment isn't accurate.

Leading Statement or Question. This technique is used to help the sender move on to additional thoughts. It is especially helpful in problem solving. The sender says, "I really don't know what to say to my family." You can say, "What are some of the things you have thought you would like to say?" This encourages the sender to list options.

Observations of Nonverbal Behavior. Being sensitive to feelings increases the amount of information available from a conversation. However, it is sometimes helpful to validate your observations. If you notice the sender frowning and sighing, you could say, "You seem to be anxious and upset." This allows the sender to verify or dispute your assessment.

Communication Barriers

Negators. "Don't worry" or "That's silly" tend to make the sender feel their concerns are not important and therefore are not to be further explored.

Accusers. "You really don't mean that" tells the sender it's wrong to feel this way and it would be best not to continue the discussion.

Assumers. "I know how you feel" can also be an enhancer, but only if you have personally experienced the same situation in the same way yourself. As this is fairly rare, this response should be used sparingly, if at all. You may say, "I have had the same operation you have," or "I have had chemotherapy, too," if that is indeed the case, but global statements are best avoided.

Directives. "You should" or "You shouldn't" take the responsibility for decision-making away from the sender and place control with you.

Cliches. "Everything will be all right" is usually the result of not knowing what to say but wanting to say something. Hand holding or supportive silence is preferable.

Value Judging. "Oh no" or "That's awful" are only appropriate if your feelings about the situation are in accordance with the sender's.

*Adapted from I CAN COPE teaching materials, American Cancer Society.

Suggested Reading

To learn more about the topics discussed in Chapter 5, the following reading material is recommended:

Borysenko, Joan. *Minding the Body, Mending the Mind.* Menlo Park: Addison-Wesley, 1987. Managing stress and anxiety and reframing life's problems into manageable proportions.

Cantor, R.C. *And a Time to Live: Toward Emotional Well-Being During the Crisis of Cancer.* New York: Harper & Row, 1978. Psychologist explores patterns of relationships and the psychological problems of cancer patients and families.

Cousins, Norman. *Anatomy of an Illness.* New York: Bantam Books, 1981. How positive emotions and relationships aid healing.

Cousins, Norman. *Head First: The Biology of Hope.* New York: Penguin, 1990. Affirming how positive emotions promote health.

Fiore, Neil A., Ph.D. *The Road Back to Health: Coping with the Emotional Side of Cancer.* New York: Bantam Books, 1986 (revised edition 1991). A cancer survivor's excellent account of the communication problems encountered by cancer patients.

Greenberg, Mimi. *Invisible Scars: A Guide to Coping with the Emotional Impact of Breast Cancer.* New York: Walk and Co., 1987.

LeShan, Lawrence. *Cancer As a Turning Point.* New York: E.P. Dutton, 1989. Recommends use of a "trained guide" in recovering from cancer

Moyers, Bill. *Healing and the Mind.* New York: Doubleday, 1993. Comprehensive and fascinating account of Moyers' PBS interviews with many professional experts exploring the mind-body connection in healing.

Siegel, B.S. *Love, Medicine and Miracles.* San Francisco: Harper & Row, 1986. An inspirational, nonscientific approach to healing and finding meaning in life.

Siegel, B.S. *Peace, Love and Healing.* San Francisco: Harper and Row, 1989. Sequel to *Love, Medicine and Miracles.*

Are We Communicating? Steps to a Terrific Doctor-Patient Relationship

1. **Always bring a written list of pertinent questions and concerns.** The list should include questions you want to ask and information you want to give. Start the list the day you make an appointment and keep it tacked up in an obvious place so you can easily add items. Encourage family members to add questions. The key word here is "pertinent." Remember, your time is limited. Use it wisely.

2. **Communication is a two-way street.** Giving information is as important as getting information. Health care professionals want to know about YOU. Consider discussing some, or all, of the following: your occupation, close relatives who have cancer, how much you already know about cancer, family problems, financial problems, work stress, hobbies and other interests, if you want children in the future, and your goals for quality of life during and after treatment.

3. **Two heads are better than one.** Ask a family member or friend to accompany you to your doctors' appointments. Choose someone who can give emotional support, who listens and remembers well, and who can think objectively. Ideally, the same person will be with you every time.

4. **Permanently record your visit on tape.** Eliminate the need to say "I forgot" when trying to recall a doctor's visit. Instead, play it back on tape. A Mayo Clinic study found that patients had to listen to a taped explanation at least

three times before understanding the whole message. The initial visit, where the diagnosis and treatment options are explained, is especially crucial.

5. **Don't say you're "just fine" unless you really are.** When health care professionals ask you how you are, they really want to know. Until you report a problem, they can't solve it. If you say "just fine" when you actually have new and frightening symptoms, that's what they'll believe. Be honest and speak up. Never withhold information out of fear.

6. **Be cooperative.** No one said having cancer is easy, and it's tempting to vent your anger at those treating you. But working as a team takes cooperation. Your health care professionals want you to succeed, even though some days it may feel like you're just one more chart on the door. One kind word often begets another, though, and smiles are contagious. Working with the professionals rather than against them yields a more productive appointment.

7. **Communicate clearly.** Words are useless if we don't understand their meaning. Doctors wouldn't think of speaking to you in a foreign language; yet sometimes they don't realize their language often sounds foreign to the layperson. Insist on hearing explanations in familiar terms. If you're unclear, repeat what you have heard and what it means to you. Keep at it until you understand.

8. **Keep to the point.** The focus of your appointment should be the cancer and its treatment, not your next door neighbor's cancer or the weather. Straying from the topic is easy, because sometimes talking about cancer isn't easy. Your list will help you stay focused.

9. **Ask, and you shall receive.** Don't ask, and you won't. Some people want to know everything about their cancer, from the exact diagnosis to the exact odds of beating it.

Others want to leave the doctor in charge; an overload of information only confuses or perhaps depresses them. Health professionals aren't mind readers. State clearly how involved you wish to be in the treatment process and what you need to know.

10. **Leave yourself an out**. The Smith Driving System teaches this as a key principle of automobile safety, but it applies to many situations in life. Your health care team is your lifeline. If any part of that team doesn't suit your standards, be prepared to find a replacement. Do you have a relationship of trust and confidence? Do you come away from appointments feeling the doctor has taken time to really listen? Are you getting state-of-the-art care? Good doctor-patient chemistry won't change the cancer, but it could improve your outlook and your understanding of the disease. Be choosy. Don't settle for second best.

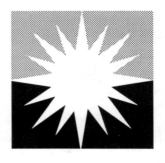

"A tiny whisper in the night . . .

Do you want to? Well, turn out the light.

Will illness keep me forever from holding her?

From knowing the smell of her skin

and the joy of enfolding her?

A fingertip stroking a cheek—

gently caressing a chin.

Illness can bring us closer . . .

we have only to begin."

Sefra Pitzele
<u>We Are Not Alone</u>
<u>Learning To Live With Chronic Illness</u>

CHAPTER SIX

Exploring Self-Esteem and Intimacy

Advertising agencies follow one key axiom—if it's sexy, it sells. New car ads feature exotic-looking women in low-cut gowns. Television and print advertisements tell us that if we wear the right fragrance, drink the right soft drinks, even chew the most flavorful gum, we will be irresistible to the opposite sex.

Sexuality Defined

After being bombarded with media inferences involving the importance of sexiness, sexuality is often viewed in very narrow terms, namely sexual performance. But sexuality is much broader than the physical and refers to all the feelings we have about ourselves as sexual beings and the ways we express those feelings to others. Sexuality and intimate relationships transcend pure physical sex. Intimacy involves not only the physical bond that exists between lovers, but the closeness of family and friends as well. And contrary to the suggestion of a popular song, *What's Love Got to Do With It*, love has a lot to do with it, starting with being able to truly love yourself.

Love of Self

Sometime in life, many people were taught that to love oneself is to be "selfish," and self-love became an unpopular notion. But until you learn to love yourself, you will have a hard time loving others or a hard time allowing others to love and accept you.

Children just naturally love themselves and believe the world revolves around them. They indulge in their own pleasures and consume the love you offer but are quite restrictive about giving love back. When parents go away, children ask, "But who will take care of me?" instead of saying, "I will miss you." As they mature into adults, emotionally healthy children learn to balance their needs against the needs of others.

Without a healthy sense of self-love, children may grow into adults who believe their needs don't matter, that they must always subordinate their needs to satisfy others. This pattern of self-denial can create tension when cancer enters the picture. Even people with a strong sense of self-worth begin to question their value. When someone says, "You look good," even though you've gained an extra 10 pounds or have lost your hair, it is hard to accept the compliment as honest.

Loving yourself is particularly hard when the "cancer is contagious" myth creates a caste of untouchables. This unfortunate misunderstanding makes many people feel unlovable and rejected, physically and socially isolated from the lives they used to lead. Being served coffee in styrofoam cups when everyone else is using china is a devastating blow to someone whose self-worth has already been shattered.

People with cancer are needy, and they deserve to have their needs met. Others in their intimate circle of family and friends sometimes have to shift gears and realize old patterns of behavior don't work anymore. The caretaker needs care. The person who has always supported the family needs support. The one who gave unconditional love now needs to be loved unconditionally. Shaking old habits is difficult; new patterns are sometimes uncomfortable. People who can make that transition are participating in the second important part of sexuality, being able to love another person.

Love of Others

People who are secure and comfortable with their own self-concept are capable of reaching out to care for others; they understand the satisfaction that comes from giving love. Selfish desires for personal happiness are tempered by a desire to also want others to be happy. Now when a loved one leaves for a few days, one can honestly say, "I will miss you," rather than "What about me?" Yet when cancer becomes a part of your life, it's easy to regress and once again become consumed with self.

Reaching out and caring for other people's wants and needs is difficult when you are preoccupied with your own health. And for now, a bit of self-indulgence is not only acceptable, it's probably necessary for emotional wellness. Family members and the person with cancer must negotiate a delicate balancing act. Maintaining independence is important, but dependency at some times is inevitable. How will everyone get their needs met? Finding an answer to that question involves the third aspect of sexuality, loving together.

Loving Together

This third dimension is usually the most rewarding aspect of sexuality for mature adults. Sexual intercourse is certainly an important part of loving together for many people. But loving together means much more than intercourse. It encompasses all the social interaction that takes place in an intimate relationship, including touching, holding, hugging, and sharing intimacies. Loving together means "being of one mind" with another human being, knowing that a certain synergy exists, where the sum of the two parts is stronger than the two standing alone.

People who love together find a natural balance between giving and receiving love. But if you were brought up with the lesson that "it's more blessed to give than to receive," sitting back and receiving the love and assistance of others may be difficult. Many people with cancer report that one of the hardest aspects of adjusting to the illness is learning how to receive love and support without feeling guilty.

Is Sexuality a Measure of Self-Worth?

Undeniably, all three of these sexual dimensions are closely linked to self-esteem in the human psyche. How we value ourselves as human beings in part stems from how lovable and attractive we believe we are to others. For instance, women's breasts have always been representative of female sexuality in the American culture. For this reason, some women go to great lengths to accentuate their breasts. Most men react to such attempts positively and thus reinforce this value. The result is that women's perception of themselves as sexual beings becomes so closely tied to their breasts that, for many, to lose a breast means losing all sexual identity.

Feelings of self-worth begin in childhood and are constantly being revised and updated. By the time we reach adulthood, the messages we have received about ourselves from parents and others close to us have helped us establish comfortable patterns of behavior. If we were brought up to believe that self-worth is largely based on our physical attributes, our patterns of sexual behavior will be linked to that belief.

Differing Views of Sexuality

Just as self-worth forms early in life, the meaning and importance of sexuality also begin at an early age. Your upbringing affects your perception of yourself as a sexual being. Some people grow up in homes where physical expression and body exposure are open and uninhibited—the bathroom door is always open. In other homes, families are more self-conscious and private about their bodies and about sexuality in general—the bathroom door is always closed.

Neither approach is right or wrong, but the chosen approach affects that person's view of sexuality. In the locker room of any health club, one can observe the results of these two styles of upbringing. Some people are unable to shower with a stranger present. Others walk around freely without clothing.

When cancer and its treatment cause bodily changes, people who have grown up with a more inhibited sexual style may find adaptation more difficult. If you dressed in the dark before a mastectomy, letting someone see your new body may prove to be a traumatic experience. People who were previously quite comfortable exposing their bodies might make this transition with greater ease.

The words families use also contribute to a person's later ability to discuss sexual issues. Many families today teach their children the proper names for their sexual organs. In more inhibited homes, euphemisms such as "down there" are used. When cancer involves sexual organs, the inhibited individuals tend to have a more difficult time discussing the cancer and how it affects them, especially if they have never discussed sexual issues before.

When cancer interrupts familiar patterns of sexual behavior, people are often forced to establish a new sexual identity. For instance, losing a breast redefines how a woman feels about herself as well as the intimacies she shares with a lover. Past attitudes and practices influence people's flexibility and help determine how comfortable they are in adapting to new sexual patterns.

The important thing to remember, regardless of your view of sexuality, is that no one is asexual. We all need and want love and usually are anxious to give love in return. For the person trying to adjust to a newly diagnosed cancer, this can sometimes be difficult. People often regress and think of themselves as unlovable; in turn, they find it difficult to reach out and love others.

One way of bringing yourself back to center is through the use of affirmations, simple statements in the present tense that "make firm" all the good and lovable things about yourself you know to be true. Cancer can temporarily turn your mind to negative thoughts. Affirmations give you a chance to replace your negative mind chatter with more positive ideas. Affirmations transform thoughts into positive attitudes and expectations. The story of *The Little Engine that Could* exemplifies the use of affirmations. By repeating the words, "I think I can, I think I can, I think I can" over and over, the engine finally convinced itself that scaling the steep hill was possible.

Adjusting to the new forms of intimacy brought on by a cancer diagnosis can be difficult. Relearning how to love yourself, then balancing the giving and receiving of love, can be difficult. But, just like the little engine, if you think you can do it, you can. At the conclusion of this chapter, you will find some simple affirmations to counteract the changes that cancer may create in terms of sexuality and self-esteem. If any of these affirmations feel comfortable, repeat them to yourself several times a day. You may be pleasantly surprised at their therapeutic effect.

Sexuality and Self-Esteem

Love of self, love of others, loving together—all are affected when cancer enters the picture. Most report changes in three general areas: changes in body image, changes in role assignments, and changes involving intimate relationships, including sexual performance.

Body Image Changes

During the time Malinda was attending I CAN COPE classes, she was enduring a rather unusual reaction from her medication. It caused her hands to peel, and the peeling skin made her hands rough and unsightly. During a hand massage exercise, she recoiled from the rest of the group. "I was so uncomfortable. I couldn't imagine anyone would want to go through that exercise with me. My hands looked and felt worse than sandpaper."

Her reaction makes one aware of how often we reach out to touch someone. A simple condition like peeling skin can cause a person to avoid reaching out and touching others at a time when human contact is more critical than ever. Continued alienation and lack of physical contact could have a devastating effect on that individual's emotional wellness.

Cancer and its treatment result in myriad bodily changes, each with its own set of difficulties. Interpersonal relationships are bound to be affected by the way people react to these changes. But learning to accept the new body image is the first step toward getting well. Affirming that the old body had to change to adjust to cancer and that the new body is more healthy is one way of learning to accept. This affirmation is difficult, and for some people, the outrage is so intense that they never succeed at total acceptance. Others may accept the changes, but they suffer from great anxiety knowing they no longer look the way they want to look.

Feeling less attractive and less lovable often causes people to retreat from both social and sexual situations in order to avoid the possibility of rejection. Unfortunately, by avoiding these opportunities for interaction, the person with cancer is also denied the positive experiences that could make them feel valued as a person.

Malinda went through the hand massage exercise even though she was uncomfortable. She found the touching soothing. "I ended up asking my partner if the roughness of my hands bothered him. I don't know if he was telling the truth or not, but he said he didn't even notice." Fear of rejection could have kept Malinda from reaching out. "I'm glad I had the nerve to do it," she said.

Both surgery and treatment can cause significant changes. Mastectomy and operations where an ostomy is required are two of the main surgical alterations of body image.

Mastectomy

As previously discussed, women's breasts in American culture have been singled out as the major symbol of female sexuality. Most women believe their womanhood would be impaired by mastectomy. About 30 to 40 percent of women who have had a modified radical mastectomy report changes in their sexual practices. A small percentage of women actually stated that they would rather die than lose a breast. It comes as no surprise that following mastectomy, many women think they are no longer sexually attractive and go through a sexual identity crisis.

Because intercourse often involves breast stimulation, mastectomy can interfere with sexual activity, and establishing new sexual patterns and habits is probably the most difficult adjustment for these women and their partners. The reported effects include an overall decrease in the frequency of sexual activity as well as specific decreases in breast stimulation and certain patterns of intercourse.

The impact varies, based on the importance both partners placed on sexual intercourse, how important the woman's breasts were within that sexual relationship, and the stability of the overall relationship before surgery. The sexual significance of the breast in the marital relationship is a particularly important factor. The partner's reaction is often more critical than that of the woman herself. If the man places a high value on physical attractiveness and the woman does not meet those standards, problems may arise. For instance, he may be reluctant to see or touch the woman's surgical scar because he finds it unattractive, even repulsive. This leaves the woman feeling unattractive and incomplete.

One way for a woman to begin overcoming problems with body image is to get comfortable with her own body. This begins by looking in the mirror and actually touching the surgical scar. You need to find out exactly how your body looks and feels without a breast. Because denial is a strong part of coping with mastectomy, some women are unable to do this right away. For several days and sometimes weeks after surgery, many mastectomy patients refuse to accept the loss of a breast. After they have been home for awhile, reality begins to set in.

Malinda spent very little time denying reality following her surgery. The doctor was very clear about what had been removed, and the weakness in her arm was proof of that. Malinda wanted to see the result. "During my first bath, I wanted to look at it. I wanted to face it as fast as I could. I looked. And I fainted. It was more than I could handle. But from then on, it got easier every time I looked." Seeing herself naked for the first time marked one of the lowest points in Malinda's cancer experience. She remembers thinking of herself as "a little invalid. Deformed. Crippled. Helpless." Yet, her upward road to recovery began with that tentative look in the mirror.

Several studies have shown that adjusting to a mastectomy may be more difficult for older women than for younger ones. Because older women are already facing the sexual implications of declining physical beauty, mastectomy often compounds the problem. This final blow to the ego can result in depression, anxiety, and insecurity. It's no wonder that 25 percent of women seek out some form of supportive counseling following surgery.

Women facing mastectomy will do better if they receive advice and support from both their doctor and their partner. The following suggestions might prove helpful:

Before surgery, ask the doctor to explain the procedure thoroughly to both you and your partner. The explanation should include the procedure to be used, the disabilities likely to result, and the rehabilitation measures that will be used to overcome the disabilities.

Seek out support ahead of time. Most hospitals offer mastectomy support groups, and Reach to Recovery is an integral part of the American Cancer Society's rehabilitation programs. Visiting with a Reach to Recovery volunteer before and after surgery has softened the impact for many mastectomy patients. It is a time of sharing with another woman who knows from first-hand experience what it is like to lose a breast to cancer.

Attempt to get your partner involved as soon after surgery as possible. A partner who changes the dressings and helps massage the arm is forced to look at the scar and become comfortable touching it.

Inquire about the possibility of reconstructive surgery. Often the prospect of plastic reconstruction of the breast offers dramatic psychological benefits. Women interested in such a procedure should discuss it thoroughly with their doctor before surgery.

Have the courage to break the silence barrier. It may be the most difficult but most productive step you can take. Your partner is wondering what to say and do. Perhaps just bringing up the topic of sexuality is difficult, so both people avoid it completely. The woman ends up feeling rejected, when in fact the loving partner is trying to be protective. Open communication is the only antidote to clearing up these misconceptions.

With time, patience, and experimentation, many women are able to overcome their self-consciousness and again feel secure and comfortable with their bodies. After reassessing their self-image and the impact of mastectomy on relationships, they may discover that femininity is not necessarily dependent on having two breasts.

Ostomy

Surprisingly, when people learn they have a cancer that involves the bladder or bowel, one of the most frequently expressed fears is the possibility of having a colostomy. Many people find even the idea of having one repulsive. Some delay consulting a doctor after seeing one of cancer's warning signals. They are more worried about the colostomy than the cancer.

Such a reaction is not unusual, considering that American society treats the topic of bladder and bowel functions as something almost unmentionable. Because most people find discussing these topics difficult and embarrassing, they avoid the subject complete-ly. With very little open discussion, it is easy to see how people conclude that there is something wrong or bad about having an ostomy. It becomes a shameful secret.

Fortunately, society is slowly becoming more informed about these topics, and attitudes are changing. We are beginning to realize that silence about important bodily functions can be destructive.

A key element in learning to adjust to an ostomy is talking with other people who are supportive and understanding. The United Ostomy Association is an organization of people of all ages who have had ostomies. They offer reassurance that often helps people feel less isolated. Many who have been through this procedure have adjusted beautifully and have resumed normal sexual activi-ties. People with ostomies and their spouses might find the follow-ing suggestions useful:

Learn to be more comfortable with your ostomy by experi-menting with the timing and with different types of appliances. Achieving a regular pattern may take some time and can be frus-trating at first. Others who have been through it can offer advice and encouragement during the early months of experimentation.

Remember that the ostomy is sutured in place and will not dis-appear back into the body. This is a fear that many people have.

Keep in mind that everyone with a bowel or bladder ostomy will have a soiling accident at some time. A good sense of humor and a good washing machine will get you through this dilemma.

For 30 minutes of lovemaking, decrease fluid intake two hours beforehand. A cummerbund is a creative way to secure the bag and allow for almost any lovemaking position.

In addition to sharing feelings with other ostomy patients, it is important to communicate your concerns to your partner as well. When you are willing to share the "secret," you and your partner will become more comfortable and feel closer.

Surgery Affecting Other Body Parts

Mastectomy and ostomy create obvious losses. You see and feel the difference from the outside. The removal of internal organs can be equally devastating. No one can see what you are missing. But once the body part is removed, a person's body image changes.

Women who have had hysterectomies report feeling an emptiness. After his lung was removed, Dick tried to picture in his mind how his body looked inside. "Just the thought of having less lung power made me tire easier," he reported. "You tend to see yourself in a new light." Even though he didn't look any different, he certainly felt different about himself.

When Bill had his kidney removed, he knew he would still be able to function normally. But lingering thoughts of the fact that "this is the only one left" make him look at life a little differently. "I take it easy on the snowmobile," he says. "And on the beer. I keep thinking that the one kidney has to do it all now."

Debbie sometimes feels like the tin man in the *Wizard of Oz*. "If I only had a brain," she laughs when she forgets something someone has said or when she can't remember a telephone number. Since her surgery, Debbie is acutely aware of the fact that part of her brain is missing. And taking the anticonvulsive medication every day for the rest of her life is a constant reminder of the fact.

Whether the body part is obvious or hidden, time and experimentation seem to be key factors in adjusting to changes in body image.

Role Changes

Because what we do is so closely tied in with who we are, a change in roles can dramatically affect self-image. People who are unable to resume their previous occupations view this as just another example of losing control. Those who have used success at work as a barometer of success in life are particularly vulnerable when cancer prompts a role change. With time on their hands and no work to make them feel productive and worthwhile, these individuals are likely candidates for depression.

Before his surgery for lung cancer, Dick was more concerned about his hands than his lungs. His doctors had warned him that the surgery would involve cutting into the ribs and muscles around his right arm. They believed he would have a long recuperation period during which he would be unable to use the right arm at all. Because his work as a highly skilled stripper in a print shop required the use of his right hand, Dick was afraid of losing his job. And losing his job meant losing his identity.

"I learned early on that it was my responsibility to support the family. When Dad died, I went right to work without even finishing high school. If I couldn't work, I wouldn't be fit to live with." Dick's wife and seven children have always depended on him. But more importantly, Dick derived most of his own self-worth from his ability to be a good provider. If cancer had robbed him of that ability, Dick would have suffered a real emotional loss.

During his six months of chemotherapy, Dick arranged his schedule so he would miss as little work as possible. He stopped at the clinic on his way to work to have his blood checked. Then he started his chemotherapy on Friday afternoon and was back to work Monday morning. Mr. Macho didn't want to let on to anyone that he was not feeling well, even though many of his weekends were spent in a drenched sweat suit only steps away from the bathroom. He made every effort to shield his family and friends from what he was experiencing.

Lou also watched her family responsibilities change. Being both a mother and a nurse, she felt most comfortable in the capacity of nurturer and caregiver. When the roles were reversed, and she was the one needing care, she felt uncomfortable. "I wanted to be the one in control. To give that control to someone else is like cutting off an arm. It's painful. It just doesn't feel right."

When the breadwinner can no longer work or the homemaker is too tired or weak to continue in that job, self-worth plummets.

"When the wife or kids would baby me or tell me to eat this or that, it really made me angry," remembers Dick. "Like I was some kind of invalid. I didn't feel like one, but that was how they treated me."

Dick's complaint is a common one. Many people express the feeling that being on the receiving end "with cancer" is different from being a receiver with another ailment, like a broken arm. Dick believes, "When you have cancer, people tend to think you are more disabled."

Over the months, Dick did a good job of hiding his illness. One weekend, an older son came home to visit while Dick was recovering from a particularly difficult round of chemotherapy. "When he saw how sick I was, he was shocked. He really had his eyes opened to what old Dad was going through! My wife Donna was never open about her emotions. But she says she screamed a lot when she was driving the van. She was 45 years old with seven kids. She felt cheated." And she was afraid. The roles in her family were shifting, and she was afraid of the possible outcome.

Dick held onto his job and did his best to protect his family from the effects of his cancer. Although cancer forced many changes on him, the fact that his work remained stable helped stabilize Dick's home life. "At the time, a steady paycheck was the best medicine I could take," he concluded.

Just as roles in the home change, social roles are also reshaped. Jim's weekly lunch with fellow employees finally became too difficult. "They all looked so good—and I knew I didn't. They would talk about their bowling or golf games. I couldn't do those things anymore. And if I wanted to talk about myself, they were uncomfortable. They wanted to hear that everything was okay. If it wasn't, they didn't want to know," he remembers.

Cancer can upset well-established social patterns. Sports activities may become too strenuous. Entertaining is difficult when food doesn't taste good or you're too tired to prepare a nice meal. Bridge or church groups are sometimes stressful when you have to excuse yourself early or you find people are treating you differently. Adapting to these social changes may take some creativity. People with cancer need to learn to put their own needs first and design social activities around those needs. The following list gives examples of ways people could customize their social life.

Learn to capitalize on what you have, not what you have lost. Malinda could see that she and her husband were growing apart. When he left Minneapolis to take a new job, she began rebuilding her social contacts. "I was blessed with the opportunity to live with Evie, and she became my friend and confidant. She knew about my cancer and she was comfortable letting me talk about it. In a way, I started a whole new life when I moved in with her."

Give yourself permission to indulge in what you enjoy. Pamper yourself with a "pamper point." When you are feeling good, reward yourself without feeling guilty. Malinda's favorite way to indulge herself was traveling. "I said to myself, 'Should I buy the expensive winter coat and boots, or should I go to California?'" She was on a plane the next week and spent a glorious, sunny week with her aunt while everyone in Minnesota was digging out from a snowstorm. We all have certain activities that give us joy—seeing a movie, lunching with a friend, fishing on a favorite lake, shopping at a special store. Pamper yourself at least once a week with something you truly enjoy. You'll feel better when you do!

Restructure your social environment based on your needs. Avoid people and places that make you feel uncomfortable or where you think others are uncomfortable around you. For many people, a cancer support group or I CAN COPE class is a great starting point for developing new interests. Malinda made many new friends through Encore, a YWCA-sponsored organization for women who have undergone mastectomies.

Communicate! Make friends and loved ones aware of the duties you can or cannot manage right now. People who continue to do as much for themselves as possible usually feel better both physically and emotionally. Don't allow others to treat you like an invalid if you don't feel like one. On the other hand, if you are feeling tired or weak and want to be pampered, make sure that is understood also. Speak up for yourself!

Changed roles are often temporary and most people adapt well when loved ones are supportive. If the home environment is not supportive, a doctor or nurse can usually put you in contact with an American Cancer Society Cansurmount volunteer who will be more than willing to offer support and friendship.

Changes in Intimate Relationships and Sexual Performance

Sexuality, broadly defined, encompasses all aspects of feeling close to the important people in our lives. It is a part of who we are and what we do. How we view ourselves as sexual beings influences our overall concept of self-worth as well as our ability to make and keep meaningful intimate relationships.

Sexuality can be expressed in many ways. It can be sharing a meal together, going for a walk, laughing over a movie, or making love. Most people have well-established patterns for intimacy. Daily habits of hugging one another or kissing morning and evening become rituals. When we are healthy, these daily interactions flow easily. Outside of normal mood fluctuations, most people are comfortable with their own style of intimate behavior.

But these familiar patterns can abruptly shift when cancer enters the picture. Cancer puts up a wall between people. Who will reach out first to remove the barrier? Honest communication becomes more important than ever. But when all parties involved are reeling from the shock of the diagnosis, it's no wonder communication becomes strained and difficult.

Communication and Sexuality

Talking about sex can be difficult. For some people, suffering in silence is more comfortable than broaching the topic and risking embarrassment or rejection. Maybe this is why several studies have concluded that better than 70 percent of all sexual communication is nonverbal. Almost all couples have ways of signaling their desires without speaking a word. One partner might wear a favorite negligee. Another may shower and use a particular after-shave lotion. Both may decide on a special dinner together or watch an erotic movie.

Even without words, the meaning is clear. We have communicated to one another our interest in making love without uttering a sound. If people have never learned to verbally clarify their sexual needs in nonstressful situations, imagine how difficult it becomes when cancer imposes an added stress. Now, when people really must talk, many don't know how.

Breaking the Silence Barrier

Doctors are also guilty of being ill at ease when it comes to discussing sexual concerns. One I CAN COPE participant's experience offers a particularly comic example. When she and her husband were at a follow-up doctor's visit, the husband was told that his wife "will have to refrain from her wifely duties for a while." The man admitted he knew exactly what the doctor meant, but since he couldn't say it, the husband wasn't about it make it any easier. Pretending innocence, he replied, "That's okay, Doc. I can just hire somebody else to do it." The doctor was forced to break the silence barrier.

Communication. Is it the universal panacea to all our sexual problems? When it comes to restoring shattered intimate relationships after a cancer diagnosis, open and honest communication is essential. But understanding how to get your message across through the use of honest, straightforward communication takes practice. Learning to be assertive instead of aggressive or passive is a good first step. An aggressive statement like, "You never talk to me or touch me anymore. What's your problem anyway?" will usually bring out a partner's defensiveness. A passive statement, like "I'm sorry I'm acting like such a baby about this" is demeaning and eliminates a person's self-respect.

"I need to be hugged and loved even though we are both upset about this thing" is a simple way of stating the situation as it is. An assertive statement like this conveys what you need without being defensive or apologetic. Even though sexual feelings and needs may change, they still are a vital part of a relationship. Partners have a responsibility to clarify how their feelings have changed and to state clearly what they need from each other.

The following statements are useful for the person with cancer to use:

- I need to be caressed and loved, but I don't think I am ready for sex tonight.

- My sexual appetite just isn't as strong anymore. But I need your closeness and support more than ever before.

- My body has changed so much, I don't feel very lovable. But that doesn't mean I don't need and want your love.

For the partner of the person with cancer, the following statements might help:

- I'm afraid of hurting you. Tell me what is comfortable for you.

- I know it's irrational, but I can't help feeling your cancer might be contagious. Let's take it slowly and give me time to adjust.

- I'm afraid you will think I'm taking advantage of you, asking you to make love when you have been through so much.

When you're not used to communicating about sex verbally, words like "I can't," or "It hurts," or "I want," or "Touch me here, but not there," or "I wish I could" are difficult to say. But clearly the old nonverbal messages are no longer adequate.

Misunderstandings are bound to occur if words are not spoken. So learn to speak up!

Specific Sexual Concerns

Besides the emotional hurdles people must scale before they can get sexually back on track, cancer is also responsible for putting up some real physical roadblocks to a healthy sexual relationship. When your body has changed because of surgery, or you are expending much of your energy to get through a rigorous treatment schedule, your sexual life may drop a few notches on your priority list.

Lack of Desire

Why does sexual activity diminish, sometimes even stop completely, after the diagnosis and treatment of cancer? Most people say it is because they feel undesirable or unworthy. "Who would want me?" asks Malinda. "For a long time, I could barely stand to look at myself, much less have someone else look at me." For women recovering from mastectomy, it is often quite difficult to resume sexual relations. The chief of psychiatry at Memorial Sloan-Kettering Cancer Center recommends that all surgeons instruct patients to return to usual sexual relations as soon as possible. In addition, she believes the woman's partner should be present when these instructions are given.

An involved and caring partner can do wonders for someone who feels undesirable and unworthy. Just as the person with cancer must face the mirror over and over again to make peace with an altered body image, the partner must also see and accept the new body. Although it may be difficult, if the partner starts by helping to change dressings and bandages after surgery, the adjustment process can start right away.

"The first time I looked at myself was the worst," recalls Malinda. "But after that, it got easier every time. I think if I could have had the courage to ask my husband to get involved right then and there, we probably could have gotten comfortable with it together."

Fatigue, worry, anger, fear, and all the other emotions that accompany a diagnosis of cancer work together to lessen a person's desire for sexual relations. In addition, surgery and treatment offer yet another group of side effects that may place love-making at the bottom of a couple's priority list. For instance, men who have had their testicles removed or who are receiving hormone therapy for prostate cancer often experience a decreased desire for sex. This usually occurs because of the reduced level of testosterone in the man's system. Testosterone, the hormone that speeds up the growth of prostate cancer cells, is also the hormone that fuels men's sexual desire.

The partner without cancer often is afraid of "catching" the disease. A husband may experience secondary impotence after his wife is diagnosed with cervical cancer. Or a wife may become disinterested after her husband is diagnosed with bladder or prostatic cancer. Even though people are repeatedly assured that cancer is not contagious, these irrational fears continue to contribute to sexual problems.

If both partners offer continued warmth and reassurance through the low times, they will keep the pilot light burning, even if the larger flame is out. Give yourself time to adjust. Making love has many more dimensions than intercourse. By touching and holding, people can remain physically close during the difficult times. This paves the way for resuming normal sexual relations when sexual desire returns.

And it will return, if you are willing to leave the door open to opportunity and change. Actress Ann Jillian, who underwent a double mastectomy and later went on to have her first baby, spoke out on her own sexual adjustment after surgery and treatment. "When women express fear of losing a breast, I point to my head and say to them, 'Ladies, your femininity is within you. Your sexiness is all up here.'" Her message is a reminder that the mind is the most potent aphrodisiac.

Malinda often uses the phrase "bloom where you are planted" when she talks about adjusting to the life changes imposed by cancer. Sexuality can bloom again too if given the right nutrients. Try to recall the early days of your relationship. Did you have special dinners together with candles and music? Did you take your time and allow for plenty of foreplay during lovemaking? Perhaps reliving these rituals will help you and your partner rediscover a mutually satisfying sexual relationship.

Fatigue

Life with cancer can be exhausting. A person's energy varies from day to day and week to week. If being sexually active is important, people can minimize exertion and maximize success by using the following suggestions:

- Plan to have sex during the time of day you feel best. If you're in the hospital, have your partner visit you during those times. Ask the nurse to hang a "Do Not Disturb" sign on your door. Hospital staff today are being instructed to be receptive to the patient's need for privacy.

- Practice self-touch as a way of relearning how to experience pleasure. Getting to know your new body and the sensations that give you pleasure, then communicating that information to your partner, will help you establish new sexual practices.

- Provide time for rest before and after intercourse.

- Avoid heavy meals and liquor before intercourse.

- Experiment with positions that require minimal exertion for the person with cancer.

- Touching, holding, kissing, sharing a back rub, or simply lying together can all be mutually gratifying alternatives to intercourse.

Pain

Pain associated with cancer or its treatment can be detrimental to sexual enjoyment. As a result of surgery, radiation, or chemotherapy, many women find they no longer produce enough lubrication for comfortable intercourse. Others experience shortening of the vagina or stenosis, a condition in which the vagina loses its elasticity. Both conditions can make intercourse painful. Men occasionally experience genital pain during sexual activity. Most often, it is caused by irritation of the prostate gland or urethra from cancer treatment. By using one of the following techniques, people can minimize the pain:

- Use water-soluble lubricants, baby oil, or vaginal gel for lubrication.

- Use a dilator to exercise and stretch the vagina.

- Take a pain medication before intercourse (not too much, however, or libido and erectile ability could be decreased).

- Try relaxation techniques before and after intercourse.

- Experiment to find the most comfortable positions, perhaps through the creative use of pillows.

Regardless of the source of the pain, the most important thing to remember is to stop when you first feel pain. Communication between partners about what feels good and what doesn't is essential.

Medication

Medication also affects a person's sexual enjoyment. Be sure to ask the doctor about potential side effects of your prescribed medicines. Some medications can temporarily interfere with the ability to have erections. Estrogen therapy may decrease a man's sexual desire. Testosterone given to a woman with breast cancer may temporarily increase her desire for sex. Other medications such as blood pressure pills, beta blockers, and muscle relaxants also can lessen a person's sexual appetite or make it more difficult to attain ejaculation or orgasm. These side effects may be temporary or permanent, depending on how long a person takes the medication. Understanding that the medication is responsible for a person's different sexual responses makes accepting those changes easier.

Inability to Experience Erections

Cancer and its treatment can interfere with a man's ability to have or sustain an erection. Surgery sometimes destroys nerves that control blood flow to the penis. Radiation treatment to the pelvis can also damage arteries carrying blood to the penis. Approximately one-third of the men receiving radiation report a change for the worse in erection capabilities. In addition, hormone therapy often makes a man feel "less like a man" because he no longer has the potent hormone testosterone flowing through his body. These feelings can result in diminished desire, which can, in turn, have an effect on the man's erection.

Although achieving an erection can be a problem, cancer treatments seldom damage the nerves or muscles involved in the sensation of orgasm. The fact that climax is still achievable makes it worthwhile to continue experimenting with sexual touching even if erection and ejaculation are not possible.

If intercourse is important and inability to have an erection truly causes a problem, ask your doctor to refer you to a sex therapist for counseling. Perhaps a professional can suggest relaxation techniques or group counseling with others who express similar problems. Or you may even consider seeing a urologist, who could assess whether or not a penile implant would be advisable.

Reproduction and Treatment—A Lethal Combination

Chemotherapy often causes some women to stop menstruating. When this happens, some feel they have lost a part of their womanhood. In most cases, this side effect is temporary and full menstrual functioning returns after a woman completes treatment.

For both men and women, radiation in the area of the reproductive organs and some chemotherapeutic drugs can cause sterility. Long-term effects usually depend on the area of exposure and the radiation dosage or on the total dosage of the chemicals. Although this sterility can be permanent, there have been instances where people have regained full reproductive capacity.

Anyone starting treatment should thoroughly discuss reproduction with a physician. Young men who hope to have a family sometime in the future might want to consider banking their sperm if they are going to be radiated in the genital area or if they are being treated with drugs that could cause sterility. Both men and women should remember that conception while undergoing any form of treatment is very risky. The risks vary with each individual. But people of child-bearing age should discuss this issue with their medical team before beginning treatment. The doctor should outline all the possible consequences of the treatment and offer suggestions for a safe, acceptable form of birth control. For instance, for some women, birth control pills are not advisable.

Open communication with the doctor is all important here, but some doctors may not initiate a discussion involving sexual issues. Young people concerned about their reproductive capacity need to make certain this topic is covered completely.

Depression and the Need for Sexual Counseling

For some people, the darkness following a cancer diagnosis becomes so deep that it's impossible to see a way out. Although anger and regret are normal and healthy, if these feelings last too long or turn into withdrawal and helplessness, professional help may be necessary. If a person's appetite for sleep, food, sex, or life in general diminish for 6 to 12 weeks or more, clinical depression should be suspected. Doctors usually recommend a combination of medication and therapy. Once the depression lifts, a person can expect to become more interested in sex.

Unfortunately, some relationships suffer when faced with the added burden of cancer. The patient may recover and learn to adjust, but the spouse cannot. At this point, the patient may end up asking a partner to "love me or leave me," sensing that the stress of a failing relationship can only make recovery from cancer more difficult. Other couples, out of guilt or insecurity, sometimes hide their true feelings and cling together in an unhealthy, hostile-dependent bond.

Sometimes it's necessary to bring in a professional counselor who can assess whether the relationship is helping or hindering the healing process of the person with cancer. Certainly some relationships are unhealthy, and the person with cancer may need help to understand the best way to deal with it. A healthy first step is to ask a doctor or nurse to recommend a qualified counselor.

Parting Tips on Getting Physical

If sex was a comfortable and enjoyable part of your life before the diagnosis of cancer, most likely it will be once again. Changes in relationships that occur while you're going through the cancer experience run the gamut. Some couples find the total life change enhances their sexual relationship. Other people are pushed apart and never regain their closeness. Somewhere in between are people who may never have given sexuality much thought and might consider it even less important now. Regardless of where you fit in this scenario, the following points should prove helpful in discovering new ways of loving one another.

Survival Overshadows Sexuality

When everything is put in perspective, just being alive comes out on top. Fighting cancer takes time and effort and involves enduring an exhausting ride on an emotional roller coaster. Fear, depression, fatigue, and anxiety will all take the wind out of your sexual sails. Taking one day at a time and being patient with yourself are important. Once the immediate crisis has passed, it is likely that your sexual interest will return.

Total Worth is Not Based on Physical Attributes

Just because you don't look the same doesn't mean anything else needs to change. You still have the same needs and desires as you had before the illness struck. Friends and loved ones will continue to love and value you—as long as you let them. Be like Malinda and "bloom where you're planted." Those who love you will be happy to nurture your new growth.

Your Most Potent Sex Organ is Between Your Ears

The mind is the most potent sex organ of all, and a cancer diagnosis can't stop your mind from creating new forms of sexual expression. Feel free to experiment and explore new ways of getting close. By building barriers around yourself or placing limitations on your sexuality, you are robbing yourself of an opportunity to discover a new sexual dimension in your life. Reach out and touch someone, and encourage them to touch you. This human contact can be a vital healing force.

Communicate. Communicate. Communicate.

Can communication be emphasized too much? Not in this case. The more talking and sharing you and your partner do, the closer you will become. At first, discussing sexual issues may seem awkward and embarrassing. Both partners may be waiting for the other one to make the first move. If too much time passes, both may start feeling rejected.

Why don't you be the one to make the first move? Start with an "I" statement like, "I never thought I'd be talking to you about sex, but I'm afraid things aren't the same, and I'd like to help us get back on track." Be open and honest about your fears and concerns. Talk about your upbringing and why you think this whole topic is so difficult. Once you and your partner begin talking, it may feel like a floodgate has been opened. A tremendous burden is lifted when people finally realize they are still loved and needed despite sexual difficulties. Honest communication makes the lifting of that burden possible.

Have Patience with Yourself and Others

Change takes patience and time. Overcoming the shock of new scars, missing body parts, and the existence of cancer itself is not an overnight process. In the beginning, take the pressure off intercourse by contracting with your partner for a specific period of abstinence from intercourse. Use this time to explore your body and rediscover your own sensuality. Then concentrate on other satisfying types of sexual expression with your partner—touching, holding, fondling, kissing, and being close. Reaching a mutually satisfying sex life will happen one step at a time.

You Don't Have to Do It Alone

If problems arise, don't hesitate to seek counseling. Your health care provider can recommend competent therapists who will work with both partners or with you alone. Because human touch is so important, and because your sexuality is closely linked to your sense of self-worth, resolving sexual concerns quickly and early is vital to your overall health. Two wonderful booklets available from the American Cancer Society, *Sexuality* and Cancer for the Woman Who Has Cancer, and Her Partner, and *Sexuality and Cancer for the Man Who Has Cancer, and His Partner*, offer a wealth of advice, both physical and emotional. Call your local American Cancer Society office and ask to receive a free copy.

Finding the Right Words

Open sexual communication sounds great, but where do you start? Who makes the first move? Who utters the first word? Perhaps the only way you will feel loved is to ask for what you need. The following words exemplify the way a person with cancer often feels. If these words apply to your life, share them with a loved one and ask for the intimacy you need.

"Can you sometimes just come and hold me? Make me feel like a child again . . . dependent again . . . taken care of again. I am not as strong as I seem. Nor am I as self-sufficient as I choose to seem. Will you let me lean on you sometimes, just a little bit? I don't want words or promises. I want the peace of a child knowing that he is loved...and cared for...and held...silently."

Suggested Reading

To learn more about topics discussed in Chapter 6, the following reading material is recommended:

Butler, Robert, and Myrna Lewis. *Love and Sex After Forty*. New York: Harper and Row, 1986. Discusses aspects of sexuality relevant to cancer patients.

Dackman, Linda. *Up Front: Sex and the Post-Mastectomy Woman*. New York: Prentice-Hall Press, 1990.

Johnson, Jacquelyn. *Intimacy: Living as a Woman After Cancer*. Toronto: NC Press Ltd., 1987. Written by a counselor who is also a cancer patient; good insight into achieving and maintaining intimacy.

Kievman, B., and S. Blackmun. *For Better or Worse: A Couple's Guide to Dealing with Chronic Illness*. Chicago: Contemporary Books, 1989.

Ornstein, Robert, and David Sobel. *Healthy Pleasures*. Reading, Mass.: Addison-Wesley, 1989.

Affirming Yourself Through Changes in Intimacy

Affirmations for Your New Body Image

Change is essential. My body is changing and I am adjusting.

I am good to my body, and my body is good to me.

I am growing stronger every day.

_____

(Write your own personal affirmation on this line.)

Affirmations for Your Changing Role

I am responsible first to myself, then to others.

What appears to be my weakness can become my strength.

I am flexible and capable of adjusting to this new role.

_____

(Write your own affirmation in this space.)

Affirmations for Your Changing Relationships

I am loved and valued for who I am.

I will accept the love of others and be glad.

I can ask for the things I need from the ones I love.

_____

(Write your own affirmation in this space.)

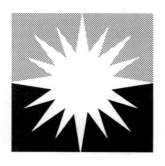

"I knew her scarcely a week,

and yet I knew her very well.

Cancer patients

have a bond

that surpasses

a healthy person's

understanding."

Cornelius Ryan
<u>A Private Battle</u>

CHAPTER SEVEN

Identifying Support Systems and Resources

Brightly colored helium balloons swing high above Malinda's mailbox welcoming the women from her Encore support group to an end-of-summer picnic. Malinda's good friend, David, dressed in a suit and tie, is busy in the kitchen preparing a batch of margaritas that he will serve in fluted champagne glasses.

Malinda, wearing pale pink to match the pink frames of her recently purchased glasses, ties more balloons to the banister before sitting down to await the arrival of her guests. A little more than a week ago, she was at the doctor's office to get "plugged in," as she calls it. At that time, she received a two-week supply of her cancer drugs, which are now being continuously fed into her system by a portable pump. But that doesn't seem to slow her down. She spent the morning cleaning patio tables and pulling weeds in Evie's expansive backyard.

"I even bought a new leather pouch to carry the chemo pack in," she says, pointing to the small burgundy purse attached to her belt. "I can't stand not being color coordinated." But her mood turns serious when she talks about the friends she has made through her association with Encore. "This picnic means a lot to me," she continues, "because these women mean a lot to me. When you're going through the whole cancer thing, you need help along the way. I found it in Encore."

People Helping People

In his book, *A Private Battle*, which chronicled his own experiences with prostate cancer, Cornelius Ryan identified the value of support systems for people with cancer when he said, "I knew her scarcely a week, and yet I knew her very well. Cancer patients have a bond that surpasses a healthy person's understanding."

People with cancer often feel alienated and talk about being utterly alone and so afraid. "Unless you've had cancer, you can't understand," Malinda says. "Other people can be helpful, but these women from Encore can relate to me. They can be supportive without pitying me."

Even when friends and family are supportive, they still don't really know what it feels like to have cancer. Consequently, sometimes the people who used to satisfy your needs aren't able to do that anymore, and you end up feeling lonely. One way to overcome the loneliness is to help one another. The people you meet at cancer-related functions understand how you feel and provide newcomers with a feeling of security and belonging they won't find anywhere else.

Self-help groups are as old as society itself. Our ancestors formed self-help organizations to get the crops in on time or get a barn raised quickly. People helping people. I CAN COPE groups are an example of people getting together in order to accomplish a common goal—learning more about cancer. But something else often takes place during the eight sessions of I CAN COPE, something most people don't really anticipate. "I came to class to learn about Hazel's cancer," John remembers. "But I soon realized that being with other people who have similar concerns helped me learn about myself, too." Group members usually feel an immediate kinship when they realize they can relax and be themselves with this group of people.

Like the others in this book, Malinda made her first peer contacts by attending I CAN COPE classes at her hospital. "Just being in a room with other people who had cancer made me feel less isolated," she remembers. "I didn't have to feel so self-conscious about my hair since the lady next to me was wearing a wig too." When the classes ended, Malinda was anxious to combine a support system with something more physical. For this reason, she chose Encore, a YWCA-sponsored group that combines water and floor exercises with education and peer support. "I joined my first Encore group because it was made up mostly of young women, much like myself. But, much to my surprise, it turned out to be a real downer. They were all very depressing. To my mind, they just took the whole business too seriously." Most of the women in Malinda's current group are much older than she is. "Age has nothing to do with it, though," she adds. "I wanted to find some women with life. With zing. These women may be older, but they definitely have that quality."

Why A Support Group?

Good Medical Care + Support + Understanding = Longer Lives

David Spiegel, M.D., professor of psychiatry at Stanford University School of Medicine, California, uncovered what many support group advocates have been saying for years—the power of group dynamics may keep people alive longer. Spiegel's group consisted of 86 women with metastatic breast cancer. All had comparable medical care, but one group had weekly supportive group therapy; the other did not. At 10-year-follow up, the three women who were still alive were from the support group. Spiegel found the group getting supportive care lived, on average, 18 months longer than the control group.

The research leading to formation of the I CAN COPE educational program was based on a similar premise. A preliminary study was conducted to determine if a structured cancer educational program could have an effect on a patient's anxiety, meaningfulness in life, and knowledge about cancer. Not surprisingly, patients who attended eight sessions of I CAN COPE reported reduced anxiety, increased knowledge about the disease, and an increased sense of the meaning of life. The study concluded that patient education is a key factor in assisting people to develop realistic expectations and attitudes toward adjusting to changes created by illness.

Before starting his support group study, Dr. Spiegel had already concluded that emotional support can significantly reduce anxiety, depression, and pain. His study was intended to see if that same type of intervention would have similar results without affecting the course of the disease. His program emphasized living as fully as possible, improving communication with family and doctors, facing and mastering fears about death and dying, and controlling pain and other symptoms. No one involved in the study, therapists and patients alike, expected that the social support would increase survival time. But it did, by a "statistically and clinically significant" 18 months. Spiegel concluded that the patients learned how to cope with stress by finding a place where they belonged, where they could express their feelings, and where they developed intense bonding with one another. They felt accepted by sharing this common dilemma of cancer.

Value of Support Groups

Victor Robinson wrote: "There is much satisfaction in work well done; praise is sweet; but there can be no happiness equal to the joy of finding a heart that understands." In addition to finding an understanding heart, what is the magic that takes place in these support systems, a magic strong enough to have an effect on physical survival? Several things come to mind:

Groups satisfy a longing to be connected. Today, the definition of family is far different from what it was in past generations. The extended family has all but disappeared, and a family today often consists of only one parent. This transition can sometimes create a feeling of isolation and loneliness. Cancer isolates people even more. Many are simply tempted to give up. Self-help groups bring people together and give them a renewed sense of belonging. Feeling connected to others increases the will to live.

Groups offer bonding through adversity. Survivors of major disasters such as plane hijackings, earthquakes, or floods often reunite to share stories of their experiences. People who survived the Holocaust continue to stay in contact with one another.

Mutual misfortune can often create a bond equal to that of ethnic or economic ties. "You get very close to people who have been down this road with you," John says. "Hazel and I feel like these group members are family now. We usually end up having supper together each week after the group meeting."

Groups turn stigma into honor. People with cancer have been labeled the new lepers, and some tell horror stories about rejection, about friends who are no longer friends, about being served meals on paper plates to avoid contamination. Facing such rejection alone is demoralizing. Sharing stories with a group bolsters your confidence. You can actually laugh at such indignities instead of crying about them.

Groups transform the helpless into helpers. When Lou decided to attend support group meetings, her intention was not to help herself. "After all the years I had been living with cancer, I thought I would be able to offer advice to others. I was pleasantly surprised to learn that they could help me just as much as I could help them." John and Hazel had a similar reaction. "When we first started out, neither of us knew much about cancer. Now, after all these years in the group, we're starting to feel like experts. Being in this group has taught us about many types of cancer, not just the cancer we had." John and Hazel were transformed from students to teachers. Today they volunteer to offer support to others who have been recently diagnosed. And, since they both remain free of cancer, their regular attendance at support group meetings is an inspiration to new members. "We're the celebrities now. I had the same cancer as Ronald Reagan. Hazel had the same cancer as his wife. And we're both healthy as horses!" After working through the initial emotions and finally accepting the cancer diagnosis as part of life, a universal sense of altruism often surfaces. This is a healthy transition, a way of turning a negative into a positive, and group experiences can perpetuate this altruism. Reaching out to others can take you out of yourself and the helplessness of your own condition and into a helping role with others. Cansurmount and Reach to Recovery are examples of ways volunteering can "make a difference" in someone else's life—and ultimately in your own as well.

Groups eliminate customary barriers. Cancer crosses all boundaries—rich and poor, black and white, male and female. Things that used to be important aren't as important anymore. How much money you make isn't as critical as how skillful you are at helping others adjust to their condition. "One time, we were asked to go to the home of one of the most powerful, influential men in our community," John remembers. "He had lung cancer, and his family hoped we could help him. It's a cinch we didn't run in the same social circles. But that didn't matter when his life was at stake."

Groups offer "back fence" knowledge and wisdom. Just as new mothers tend to trade child-rearing tips over morning coffee, support groups offer people with cancer a chance to share their own tried-and-true ideas with one another. "Over the years, we have seen many people go through chemotherapy. It seems like everyone has at least one helpful idea for making it more comfortable. People grab onto those ideas and use them. And most of the time, they are things you won't hear at the doctor's office or read in books."

Because eating properly during chemotherapy treatments is often a problem, people usually suggest foods that have worked well for them. For Bill, it was potatoes. To help him get enough calories every day, Lothair's wife, Ruth, made a special milkshake using eggs and fresh fruit. Malinda chewed on Starburst candy to make her mouth feel better. These folksy bits of advice on "what tastes good and what doesn't" won't reach the medical books. But they are practical suggestions being offered by someone who has "been there." Such commonsense ideas are usually taken just as seriously as the advice offered by the professionals. "The doctors mean well," John stresses, "but they haven't been in your shoes. And they're so busy with your medical needs, they don't have time to baby you. Support groups start where the doctor leaves off."

Groups allow powerful emotions to be expressed. A lot of hugging and crying goes on within a support group. People do this openly without shame or discomfort, and the loving support provides inspiration and bonding. The most successful way of comforting a hurt child is to hold them close. People with cancer are hurting, too. The touch of someone who cares is a powerful tool in the healing process. "When new people join the group, they sometimes spend half the time crying," Hazel observes. "They often admit it's the first time they've really cried since they learned about the cancer."

From crying to laughing, hugging to hating, talking to silence, just being in a supportive, understanding group environment can bring out pent-up emotions. Many are surprised to discover how much emotion they've been holding in.

Finding the Right Support Group

Each support group has its own unique personality. That personality is based on the combined personalities of the members and on the attitude of the person leading the group. As Malinda discovered, all support groups are not equal. The young women in her first group didn't suit Malinda's personality and style. But she continued looking. It would be a mistake to give up on support groups just because the first one you attend makes you uncomfortable.

Some people naturally gravitate toward organized groups Others are more private and find it difficult to warm up to a bunch of strangers. After her surgery for breast cancer, John's wife, Hazel, hesitated when he suggested attending I CAN COPE education classes. "John is more outgoing than I am and is comfortable in almost any group," Hazel says. "I was nervous about going someplace where I would have to talk about my cancer."

But they went. And when the eight classes were over, John and Hazel continued to attend a weekly support group at the hospital. Four years later, John's colon cancer was diagnosed. "Being a part of that group for four years made it much easier to adjust to John's diagnosis," Hazel admits.

People with cancer have learned the value of time. For this reason, they usually cut through the barrier of small talk and zero in on truly essential issues. One I CAN COPE instructor and support group facilitator talks about being constantly amazed at the honesty within groups.

"These people discuss very stressful, very personal issues within the first couple of meetings. Many of us are literally strangers to them, but they sense that they don't have time to waste on preliminaries. With that kind of group dynamic, you feel like something has really been accomplished when the hour is over." For this reason, most groups have very strict rules involving confidentiality. "What is said here stays here," she stresses. "We want our group to be a place where people can ventilate their feelings without fear of having them repeated."

Financial and Legal Resources

When Jim learned his cancer had metastasized to his liver, he was upset and yet not depressed. But the first two treatments were not very effective in slowing the cancer's growth. The doctor suggested getting his affairs in order. "That was depressing," Jim admits. "But it made me realize that all of us are going to die sometime. And it's smart to get those things done even if you're not sick."

"Jim wanted to make arrangements for his funeral right away," Shirley adds. "I told him we might as well do it for both of us. Something could happen to me, too. Then, when everything was settled, I told him, 'Now that we've taken care of our death, let's get on with the business of living.'"

Living is a business. And included in the business of living are a home, a job, a family, bank accounts, personal property, pension plans, insurance policies. The list seems endless. And if someone dies without having a clear accounting of all these items, it can be a nightmare for the grieving survivors.

Addressing practical concerns is difficult when you're in the process of fighting for your life. Yet adequate preparation will undoubtedly minimize any legal or financial difficulties in the future. The next few pages offer brief suggestions on a variety of issues that should be discussed frankly with all family members. Professional legal counsel may be required on many of the items. It is well worth the investment.

Personal Inventory

Look for the sample "Personal Inventory Form" at the end of this chapter. Simply filling out this form is a valuable first step toward getting organized. Copies of certain records and documents should be put in one place where your family can find them. This can be done by placing everything in a brown envelope, clearly marking the outside, and putting it in a place known to your family. Originals of one-of-a-kind documents (wills, real estate titles, etc.) should remain in a safe deposit box. Make copies of these documents to include in the envelope.

Once you have done all the preliminaries, schedule a family conference and share all the information with everyone. Knowledge is power, and everyone should end up feeling more comfortable after discussing this vital information.

Medical Insurance

Dealing with insurance becomes a major part of dealing with cancer. In most instances, if you were not covered by a health insurance plan when your diagnosis was made, it will be difficult to obtain coverage now. Most insurers require a treatment-free period before offering coverage. If you are currently covered, it is probably through group coverage offered by your employer or by Medicare.

Private Insurance Plans

If you have private insurance or are part of a group plan provided by your employer, your first step is to get a current copy of the plan booklet and examine it to determine exactly what is covered. The employee benefits department of most companies have this booklet.

Look for the following points in your plan:

Understanding Your Insurance Plan

- Amount of the deductible before the plan begins to pay.

- Number of hospital days and amount paid per day.

- Surgical and anesthesia costs.

- Percentage of charges carrier will pay (normally in the 80 to 100 percent range).

- Reimbursement for second opinions.

- Total dollar amount payable for your lifetime.

If you are no longer working but are still covered by your previous employer's plan, you are probably responsible for the premium payments. It is crucial you pay on time to avoid having the policy lapse.

Some plans have a time limit within which you must notify the company of your intent to file a claim. Be sure you understand the claim form procedure. If you are filing your own claim, keep a file with plenty of claim forms and submit them as soon as you have a bill. If the hospital or doctor's office submits the claim, ask to receive copies of all their paper work.

When in doubt, file a claim. If the claim is refused, and you believe the item should have been covered, don't take no for an answer. Begin by voicing your protest to the claims department. If this is not successful, continue up the corporate ladder within the insurance company until you are satisfied with their answer.

In all insurance matters, make it a habit to keep good records. Buy a two-pocket folder and label the front "Insurance Matters." On the left side, store your plan booklet along with blank insurance forms and envelopes. On the right side, keep copies of your submitted claims and all correspondence you have received from the company.

Long-Term Insurance Options

Cancer survivors need insurance for life, and sometimes finding long-term coverage is difficult. If you are able to return to work after cancer treatment and are still covered by your company's insurance policy, plan carefully before you consider changing jobs. Don't leave a job with insurance benefits until you have a new job with good coverage. Sometimes you're even better off taking a new job at less salary if the insurance coverage is better.

If you leave your old job, you have the right to convert to an individual policy. The Comprehensive Omnibus Budget Reconciliation Act (COBRA) protects you for 18 months by allowing you to continue buying coverage through your employer. After the 18-month period expires, you will need to find another insurance option. You might consider the following avenues.

Convert your group policy to a permanent individual plan. Be careful, however, since benefits may be greatly reduced and the premium greatly inflated.

Find employment with the biggest company you can. Look for an employer with 300 plus employees.

Check with your state Blue Cross/Blue Shield plan. Each state varies, but in some states, Blue Cross/Blue Shield must sell you insurance regardless of your health. Check the waiting period for pre-existing illness.

Call the State Insurance Commissioner's Office. Some states have high-risk plans or can offer other suggestions.

Buy an Excess Major Medical (Catastrophic Major Medical) Policy. This is in addition to your Basic Major Medical (Comprehensive) Plan. The deductible is very high, after which the plan pays 100 percent. It's relatively inexpensive and often is available through fraternal or professional association memberships.

Check for open enrollment with an HMO. Remember you must use their doctors and hospitals.

Medicare

The federal government is responsible for the Medicare program, which is funded by Social Security taxes. Although Medicare does provide protection against large health care costs, it does not cover everything. People who are 65 years of age or older are eligible for Medicare benefits. In some instances, people under the age of 65 also qualify for Social Security benefits. If you have questions regarding eligibility, call your local Social Security Administration office.

Medicare's Hospital Insurance (Part A) helps pay for many of the costs associated with the first 90 days of inpatient hospital care. Deductibles do apply, however, so it would be wise to check the current plan to see how much out-of-pocket expense will be required. Everyone eligible for Social Security benefits is automatically covered by the hospital insurance.

Medicare's Medical Insurance (Part B) covers doctors, outpatient services, home health care, and other medical services and supplies. This insurance is voluntary and requires payment of a premium. Congress decides the amount of the premium, which is based on a percentage of the program cost. In addition, there is a yearly deductible and payments are limited to 80 percent of approved charges.

Medicare coverage is discussed completely in the booklets *Your Medicare Handbook and Guide to Health Insurance for People with Medicare.* Both booklets are free and can be obtained by calling your local Social Security office. Look in the white pages under U.S. Government, Department of Health and Human Services. If it is convenient, visiting your Social Security Office to pick up the booklet may be more productive. They are often swamped with telephone requests, which can result in a delayed response. By making a personal visit, you will be assured of getting their most recent printed material.

Trusts and Wills

Establishing a trust is a complex procedure and usually is only considered by people with large estates who want a bank to manage that estate for them. A will is a legal document that allows you to distribute your assets exactly as you choose. Without a will, state statutes decide how assets are distributed. And many times, the disposition is far different from what you might have chosen. A will is especially important if you have children under the age of 18. The will should name a guardian and set up trust funds for the children. If both parents should die without a will, the courts would determine custody of the children and distribute the assets.

Because a will is a legal document, it should be drawn up by an attorney. Each state has different laws regarding wills. If you had a will drawn up in another state, it should be reviewed at your current residence. Family situations change constantly. What may have been an appropriate disposition of your estate several years ago may not pertain today. Be sure to review your will if your circumstances have changed. You can change your will at any time simply by adding a codicil. Always have an attorney make any necessary adjustments.

Living Wills

A Living Will simply states that you want the right to die with dignity by having a natural death, and it makes it possible for you to state your wishes now when there is no doubt about your mental competency. If you don't wish to be kept alive artificially or to have heroic measures used to sustain life, you should seriously consider a Living Will.

In many states, certain conditions apply before a Living Will is considered valid. Usually, the attending doctor needs to verify that the individual has a condition that is terminal and incurable and that information should be confirmed by another doctor. The Living Will form can be obtained from any attorney, must be witnessed and signed in accordance with state law, and must be certified by a notary public. Witnesses cannot be related to the person making the Living Will.

Can you change your mind once you have signed a Living Will? Yes, you may revoke a Living Will by destroying the original and all copies or by simply communicating your intent to revoke the will to all interested persons.

Power of Attorney

Paperwork is a major headache for the person with cancer and family members. Just coping with cancer and its treatment is a big enough challenge. But when paperwork starts piling up, the challenge looms even larger. If managing your affairs becomes too burdensome, you can appoint someone to manage them for you by granting that person power of attorney. That person can then make legal and financial decisions on your behalf. It lasts until you revoke it or you become incapacitated.

A durable power of attorney extends the terms of the standard power of attorney so that it lasts until your death or until you revoke it. Of course, it must be made while you are mentally competent. Unlike the regular power of attorney, it doesn't expire if you become incapacitated.

Some states now have a durable power of attorney for health care. This allows someone else to make important decisions regarding your health care. If you are considering a Living Will, it would be wise to also assign a durable power of attorney for health care to someone who then would be responsible for managing medical decisions so they follow your directives. State laws vary on all these legal documents. Consult a lawyer who is familiar with your state's legal requirements.

Bank Accounts

If you and your spouse hold a bank account in joint tenancy, both people have access to the account. If one person dies, that access remains unchanged. If you have accounts in your name alone, the money in that account would be distributed according to your will or by the courts in the absence of a will. In either case, it could take some time before those funds became available. You should consider this in planning for a family's immediate financial needs. Just cashing or depositing a spouse's Social Security check could be a problem if you don't already have automatic deposit. Assigning power of attorney to a family member would make managing all these funds somewhat easier.

Safe Deposit Box

Personal records should not be stored in a safe deposit box where only one person has access. If you were to put your will in a box rented solely in your name, it would be difficult for anyone to get at that will in the event of your death. Heirs will have access to the contents of the box only after the will is executed.

Insurance Policies

Before payment can be made on any insurance policies, the original copy of the policy must be presented along with a death certificate. It is wise to review the designation of beneficiaries on your policies if you have not done so lately. Circumstances may have changed since the policies were first initiated. Some mortgages, car loans, and installment loans have a provision by which the insurer automatically repays the balance due in the event of your death. Look over all policies and make a note of any that offer this provision.

Pension Plans

Most people today are covered through their employer by a pension or profit-sharing plan. You should take the time to acquaint loved ones with all the provisions of that plan. A family discussion now will pave the way for survivors to obtain maximum benefits. For instance, would payments continue to your surviving spouse? Does the pension system pay death benefits? Does your spouse have the necessary information to make the appropriate claims? If these are the kinds of things you always took care of without including your spouse, they could easily be overlooked by a grieving family.

Social Security Benefits

To receive Social Security survivor benefits, you must apply at a Social Security office. You need to have certain documents on hand to complete an application. Call your local Social Security office and ask to be sent the booklets describing all the details.

Veterans Benefits

By checking with your local Department of Veterans' Affairs, listed in the white pages under "U.S. Government," you can learn the benefits to which you are entitled. Even if your cancer is not service related, you may be eligible for certain benefits, especially if your income is limited. A booklet entitled *Federal Benefits for Veterans and Dependents* is available for a small fee from the Superintendent of Documents, U.S. Government Printing Office, Washington, D.C. 20402. It explains the health, hospitalization, disability pension, life insurance, and other benefits available. You may qualify for certain types of inpatient or outpatient care, based on financial need. Disability pensions are possible if you served during wartime and are totally and permanently disabled.

Job Discrimination

Today, the American Cancer Society estimates that there are eight million cancer survivors in the U.S. A National Institutes of Health report shows 80 percent of cancer patients eventually return to work. Yet one of every four people who have cancer faces employment problems or encounters some form of job discrimination based on health history. Why? Employers and coworkers still hold on to old cancer myths—cancer is contagious, cancer survivors can't work hard, or the person is going to die.

Most cancer survivors are anxious to get back to work and resume a normal life. Most employers are fair and do all they can to accommodate the person with cancer. But in some cases, people find they can't get their old jobs back. Or they are denied promotions or raises when they return. They may be forced to work in unpleasant conditions. What legal recourse do they have?

National Coalition for Cancer Survivorship

Although the civil rights movement originally was confined to discrimination based on race, religion, national origin, and sex, the collective voice of more than 8 million cancer survivors is beginning to be heard. The National Coalition for Cancer Survivorship (NCCS) was formed for the purpose of organizing local survivorship groups into a national network. Their goal was to promote an understanding of cancer survivorship and unite various survivor groups and patient advocate programs into a single survivorship movement. Today the coalition's overall mission is to disseminate information about living through cancer and paying for it, as well as to argue for health care reform that benefits cancer survivors.

One of the first items on the agenda of the NCCS was to expand job opportunities by prohibiting employment decisions based solely on health status instead of individual qualifications.

Family and Medical Leave Act

The Family and Medical Leave Act (FMLA) now requires employers with 50 or more employees to provide up to 12 weeks of unpaid, job-protected leave for family members who need time off to address their own serious illness or to care for a seriously ill child, parent, or spouse. During the leave period, the employers must continue to provide benefits.

If you are looking for a new job, the Rehabilitation Act of 1973 outlaws discrimination based on handicap; it protects healthy cancer survivors from job discrimination and applies to all employers receiving federal assistance. Employers covered by this act include federal, state, and local governments; most schools and universities; and institutions receiving federal grants.

Americans With Disabilities Act (ADA)

This act now protects more cancer survivors than the Rehabilitation Act because it covers private employers who don't receive federal funds. If your rights under the ADA are violated, you can file a complaint with the Equal Opportunities Commission, listed in the white pages under "U.S. Government."

When you are looking for work, remember that it is illegal for an employer to require you to disclose your medical history until after they have agreed to hire you. And you can't be required to submit to a physical exam designed to screen out a disability like cancer. To learn about specific laws in your state, contact your local American Cancer Society office or telephone the National Coalition for Cancer Survivorship at 1-301-650-8868. If you believe your employer is discriminating against you based on your illness, contact the American Civil Liberties Union, a legal aid group in your area, or the NCCS.

Employment Considerations for Survivors

- Look for Equal Opportunity Employers.

- Look for government contractors who are covered by Section 503 of the Federal Rehabilitation Act.

- Nearly all schools, colleges, hospitals, and institutions are covered by Section 504 of the Federal Rehabilitation Act.

- Ask when you apply if the company is covered by any of these programs.

Health Care Resources

Bridging the gap between hospitalization and home can be a frightening adjustment. Fortunately, several options are available that make that transition easier, including home health care and hospices. The American Cancer Society, in particular, offers a variety of equipment and services, most of which are available at little or no cost to the user.

Resources of the American Cancer Society

Cancer Response System (CRS). When you or someone close to you has cancer, not understanding what is going on can be frightening. The Cancer Response System is national toll-free hotline you can call to learn more about a specific type of cancer, its detection, treatment, and rehabilitation. CRS also provides the name of your local ACS chairperson, who can refer you to local services and support groups. Just call 1-800-ACS-2345.

Sickroom Equipment. Many pieces of equipment are available for loan to private homes through ACS and may be borrowed for as long as needed for the care and comfort of the person with cancer. Items available include hospital beds, siderails, wheelchairs, walkers, canes, lambs wool, urinals, bedpans, and commodes. Insurance, Medicare benefits, or both are used when appropriate.

Medical Dressings and Gift Items. Hair loss is a common problem. In many areas, the ACS supplies Kathy Kaps (attractive head scarves), which are a welcome solution to this problem. The ACS also offers suggestions on finding wigs. In addition, they can provide dressings, sponges, gowns, slippers, and many other items needed during recuperation.

Road to Recovery. Sometimes the biggest obstacle to recovery can be just getting to and from the treatment center. ACS now takes this worry away by providing transportation through what is sometimes called the Road to Recovery program. This service provides volunteers to drive patients to and from treatment centers. By contacting your local ACS office before the time the actual service is needed, transportation can almost always be arranged.

Home Health Care

The rapidly changing face of health care has shifted the emphasis away from long-term hospitalization toward quality home health care. By making use of the many services provided by home health agencies, people with cancer and their families are relieved of day-to-day responsibilities that can become overwhelming.

With the approval of their physician, people with cancer can now receive a variety of home care services and treatments, including total parenteral nutrition, tube feeding, chemotherapy, pain management, antibiotics, or a combination of several treatment regimens. Some people only need help with housekeeping chores. Others require some type of nursing assistance. People who have had surgery may need physical or speech therapy. Some prefer to have their chemotherapy at home instead of going into the hospital or clinic.

If you think you need one or more of the above services, the easiest place to start is with the social worker at your local hospital. The local chapter of the American Cancer Society also should have a list of home health agencies. Remember that an integral part of successful home care is the bond of trust between the provider and the patient. Whether the care is given by a family member or a home care service, be sure you have faith and confidence in your provider. For more information on home care, contact the Foundation for Hospice and Home Care, the National Association for Home Care, or the Visiting Nurse Association. Addresses and telephone numbers are listed later in this chapter.

Hospice

The word "hospice" originally referred to the safe refuge offered weary travelers and pilgrims in medieval times. At the end of a long day's journey, they could look forward to being fed and cared for in the warmth of a way station—or hospice. Our current concept of hospice as a place of refuge for terminally ill patients began in England and was introduced to the United States in 1974. Today, hospice programs provide specialized care and support for people with limited life expectancies and their families.

Although hospice was originally conceived as an inpatient program, under the current health care system, most hospice patients receive care and support at home. Today thousands of hospice programs are available nationwide. In the United States, approximately a quarter of a million terminally ill patients and their families receive hospice care every year, most of which is provided in the comfort of their own home environment.

When treatment is no longer curative, hospice provides the opportunity for a person to live each day as fully and completely as possible in an atmosphere of home and family. A team of professionals provides physical care, psychological support, comfort, and hope.

Lou chose a hospice program when she became so weak she was spending most of her time either on the couch or in bed. A visiting nurse from the hospice service started coming to Lou's home daily to tend to her physical care and make sure her medications were being administered properly. "From the very beginning, my nurse Marlene treated me like I was a member of her own family," Lou recalls. "She was very caring and concerned. She also acted as a liaison between me and the doctor, so he had a running report on my condition."

After more than 20 years of living with cancer in a strong and cheerful manner, Lou agreed it was time to leave her own home and adopt hospice as a new home. Always a positive, dignified woman, Lou wanted to be in an environment that mirrored her personality. "We couldn't praise hospice enough," Ingvar concluded when asked if they were both satisfied with Lou's care. "The staff bent over backwards to satisfy the family's needs. When our two boys arrived, we were told we could all stay right in the hospice overnight free of charge whenever we want. And the food they serve is out of this world."

Hospice emphasizes treatment of the person, not the disease, and allows people an opportunity to regain some control by involving them in the planning process. In addition to making the patient comfortable through proper pain medication and relief from unwanted symptoms, hospice also strives to offer emotional support to both patient and family. The hospice team, made up of physicians, nurses, social workers, psychologists, clergy, and specially trained volunteers, evaluates the family and plans a program to suit each family's particular circumstances. For instance, in some families, religion becomes an important part of their hospice experience. Others want little mention made of religion. The team is sensitive to such differences.

Hospice can accept for care only people who are considered terminally ill. This may be the first time many families have actually faced the thought of losing a loved one. The hospice team is trained to offer counseling and support as people attempt to come to terms with this reality.

A portion of the hospice expenses are often covered under private insurance plans, Medicare, or Medicaid. For more information on exactly what is covered through Medicare or for the location of Medicare-certified hospice programs, get in touch with the National Hospice Organization by calling 1-800-658-8898.

Resources for Additional Information

When giving information to people with cancer, it is difficult to know where to draw the line. How much do you want to know about individual types of cancer? About treatment facilities in your location? About support networks you can tap? About helpful books and pamphlets? The following paragraphs suggest other places you can look for this specific information.

American Cancer Society

Under the umbrella of the American Cancer Society (ACS), more than 2 million people operating out of 57 separate divisions work together to fight cancer. Their services include information and patient education, transportation, equipment loan or rental, dressings, and volunteer visitors programs.

The ACS receives no government support and relies on donations from the public to fund its services. Volunteers make up the heart of ACS. Without the time, energy, and skills of a large corps of volunteers, ACS could not offer such a wide variety of services. What follows is a list of many of the programs ACS volunteers provide. If you are interested in one of these services, check the telephone directory for your nearest ACS office. If you can't find one, contact the national office at 1599 Clifton Road NE, Atlanta, GA 30329-4251, 1-800-ACS-2345.

Volunteer Visitor Programs

Reach to Recovery. Success breeds success. If you are just starting down the road to recovery after breast surgery, few things are as uplifting as talking with someone who has been in your position and made a successful recovery. The Reach to Recovery program of the American Cancer Society is a one-on-one visitation program for women who have breast cancer. It provides information and support to a newly diagnosed patient by someone who has been through the breast cancer experience herself—the Reach to Recovery volunteer visitor. All Reach to Recovery volunteers are carefully trained by the ACS to help a breast cancer patient meet the physical, emotional, and cosmetic needs related to her disease and its treatment.

Ostomy Visitor Program. Trained volunteer visitors assist patients who have had bowel or bladder surgery. They offer emotional support and practical advice on adjusting to life with an ostomy. The United Ostomy Association cooperates with the ACS in providing this program.

Laryngectomee Clubs. Trained visitors offer support and education both before and after surgery. The local member clubs of the International Association of Laryngectomees provide education as well as continued social and emotional support.

Cansurmount. The Cansurmount program is a one-on-one visitation program for cancer patients and is not site-specific like Reach to Recovery. Trained volunteer visitors who have already had cancer are matched with newly diagnosed cancer patients. The volunteer provides both emotional support and practical information on a short-term basis. These volunteers know how you feel because they have been in your shoes.

Education and Information

I CAN COPE. This book provides you with the basic format of the eight sessions that make up the I CAN COPE educational program. But attending I CAN COPE classes allows patients and their families to receive the most current information from health professionals in their area. It also affords people an opportunity to meet other families who are learning to live with cancer. Getting out and socializing with others is sometimes equally as important as the information presented in these classes.

Look Good...Feel Better. This program is designed to help women recovering from cancer deal with the unpleasant side effects of cancer treatment such as dry skin, loss of hair, etc. By gaining control over these side effects, they discover that looking good can actually help them feel better. This program is co-sponsored by the Cosmetic, Toiletry, and Fragrance Association and the National Cosmetology Association.

ACS Publications. The American Cancer Society provides many publications free of charge. By calling your local ACS office, you can receive a brochure on each individual type of cancer. They also provide many useful booklets, including the following:

- *Answering Your Questions About Cancer*
- *Cancer Facts and Figures*
- *If You Find a Lump in Your Breast*
- *Listen with Your Heart: Talking with the Cancer Patient*
- *Nutrition for Patients Receiving Chemotherapy and Radiation Treatment*
- *Questions and Answers About Pain Control*
- *Sexuality and Cancer for the Man Who Has Cancer, and His Partner*
- *Sexuality and Cancer for the Woman Who Has Cancer, and Her Partner*
- *Talking with Your Doctor*
- *What is Chemotherapy?*

National Cancer Institute

The National Cancer Institute is funded through the U.S. Department of Health and Human Services. The Cancer Information Service is a nationwide telephone service for cancer patients and their families and friends, the public, and health care professionals. The staff can answer questions in English or Spanish and can send free National Cancer Institute booklets about cancer. They also know about local resources and services. One toll-free number—1-800-4-CANCER (1-800-422-6237)—connects callers with the office that serves their area. Phones are answered Monday through Saturday by trained, certified volunteers and professional staff.

PDQ

By calling the Cancer Information Service, you can now gain access to a computerized information service called Physician Data Query or PDQ. This service provides both doctors and patients with access to up-to-date cancer treatment information. Through the PDQ, you can learn about cancer staging, appropriate options at any given stage of cancer, and your prognosis for survival. You can also receive information about the closest treatment center and what physicians in your area are offering the most current state-of-the-art treatment. This cancer information file is updated monthly based on the recommendations of 29 prominent doctors with expertise in treating cancer.

To request a computerized PDQ, contact the Cancer Information Service and have the following information in front of you:

- Your diagnosis, including type and stage of cancer.

- Where the primary cancer is located.

- The cell type.

- Name, address, and telephone number of your doctor.

Because the material you will receive is written in technical terms best understood by a doctor, you should have the report mailed to your doctor. The two of you can then sit down and go through the report together. Once the doctor has explained everything, treatment options can be discussed.

The PDQ also lists approximately 1,300 clinical trials being used to evaluate new approaches to cancer treatment. If you're interested in a clinical trial, work with your doctor using PDQ to find the appropriate choice.

National Cancer Institute Publications

The National Cancer Institute (NCI) publishes a series of booklets called *What You Need to Know*. The booklets discuss almost every type of cancer. When requesting one of these booklets, be sure to specify the exact type of cancer. The following excellent booklets are also provided by NCI and can be obtained by calling 1-800-4-CANCER. You may also want to ask for an NCI publication list; it includes all of NCI's booklets.

- *Advanced Cancer: Living Each Day*
- *Answers to Your Questions about Metastatic Cancer*
- *Chemotherapy and You: A Guide to Self-Help During Treatment*
- *Eating Hints: Recipes and Tips for Better Nutrition During Cancer Treatment*
- *Facing Forward: A Guide for Cancer Survivors*
- *Questions and Answers about Pain Control (published jointly with the American Cancer Society)*
- *Radiation Therapy and You: A Guide to Self-Help During Treatment*
- *Taking Time: Support for People with Cancer and the People Who Care about Them*
- *When Cancer Recurs: Meeting the Challenge Again*

Other Helping Organizations

American Bar Association
750 Lakeshore Drive
Chicago, IL 60611
(312) 988-5000
May link cancer patients with an attorney in their area who is familiar with cancer-related issues. People can also call their local Lawyer's Referral Service.

Bone Marrow Transplant Family Support Network
P.O. Box 845
Avon, CT
(800) 826-9376
Offers counseling and support for people considering or undergoing bone marrow transplant.

R.A. Bloch Cancer Foundation, Inc.
4410 Main Street
Kansas City, MO 64111
(816) 932-8453
Founded by Richard Bloch, a cancer survivor, this foundation utilizes a multidisciplinary professional panel to give free second opinions on an individual's cancer treatment. By calling this telephone number, you can also access the Cancer Hotline, which provides "phone mates" for people just diagnosed. The phone mate is someone who has recovered from a similar type of cancer.

Cancer Care, Inc.
1180 Avenue of the Americas
New York, NY 10036
(212) 366-2223

Provides information and support for parents of children with cancer. Puts out quarterly newsletters with information on childhood cancer.

Candlelighters Foundation
7910 Woodmont Avenue, Suite 460
Bethesda, MD 20814
(800) 366-2223
Provides information and support for parents of children with cancer. Publishes quarterly newsletters with information on childhood cancer.

Corporate Angel Network (CAN)
Westchester County Airport Building I
White Plains, NY 10604
(914) 328-1313
Arranges free transportation on corporate aircraft for cancer patients receiving treatment at centers approved by the National Cancer Institute.

Encore
YWCA of the United States
726 Broadway, 5th Floor
New York, NY 10003
(212) 614-2827
Peer support, exercise, and rehabilitation for postmastectomy patients.

Foundation for Hospice and Home Care
519 C Street NE
Washington, DC 20002
(202) 547-6586
Provides low-cost publications and general consumer advice.

Leukemia Society of America
600 Third Avenue
New York, NY 10016
(212) 573-8484
(800) 955-4572 (information hotline)
Supplies information on medical, psychological, and financial help for patients with leukemia, Hodgkin's disease, and lymphoma. In some cases will provide financial help of up to $750 for outpatient costs not covered by other sources.

Make Today Count
101/2 So. Union Street
Alexandria, VA 22314
(703) 548-9674

A peer support network with more than 200 local chapters around the world. These groups offer emotional support to people with all types of life-threatening illness and are not limited to cancer alone. This self-help organization often depends on the buddy system to assist people in improving the quality of life, despite chronic illness.

*National Association for Home Ca*re
519 C Street NE
Washington, DC 20002
(202) 547-7424

Represents all home health care agencies in the U.S. for legislative and regulatory issues. They will provide a booklet entitled "How to Select a Home Care Agency."

National Alliance of Breast Cancer Associations (NABCO)
1180 Avenue of the Americas
Second Floor
New York, NY 10036
(212) 221-3300

Provides information on educational materials about breast cancer, promotes affordable and accessible detection and treatment, advocates for laws benefiting women with breast cancer, and serves as voice for their rights and concerns.

National Coalition for Cancer Survivorship
1010 Wayne Avenue, 5th Floor
Silver Spring, MD 20910
(301) 650-8868

With a goal of enhancing the quality of life for cancer survivors, this organization actively works for health care reform and strives to promote an understanding of cancer survivorship, publishes the Cancer Survivors Almanac of Resources.

National Hospice Organization
1901 N. Moore Street, Suite 901
Arlington, VA 22209
(800) 658-8898

Provides referrals, information, and support regarding services for the terminally ill; information will benefit professionals, volunteers, and the general public.

United Ostomy Association
36 Executive Park, Suite 120
Irvine, CA 92714
(714) 660-8624
(800) 826-0826

Sponsors hospital and home visits by recovered ostomy patients to assist in rehabilitation through moral support and education. They publish Ostomy Quarterly for members and they support efforts for improved equipment, supplies, and management techniques.

US TOO
P.O. Box 7173
Oakbrook Terrace, IL 60181
(708) 627-6834

Support, information, and educational meetings for men with
prostate cancer and their family members.

Visiting Nurse Associations of America
3801 E. Florida Avenue, Suite 900
Denver, CO 80210
(800) 426-2547

Provides skilled nurses, therapists, and home care aides at centers throughout the United States.

Y-ME Breast Cancer Support Program, Inc.
18220 Harwood Avenue
Homewood, IL 60430
(708) 799-8228 (24-hour hotline)
(800) 221-2141

Information and support, plus a wig and prosthesis bank for
patients with breast cancer.

United Cancer Council
1803 No. Meridian Street
Indianapolis, IN 46202
(317) 923-6490

Provides services, medications, prostheses, and sometimes can
provide direct financial assistance.

Additional Reading Material

Some people want a lot of concrete, factual information. That's why several book titles covering factual material are listed at the end of each chapter of this book. Many of these books are available at your local library.

But a well-rounded cancer education should also include a few books that are written from the personal or inspirational perspective, since the lessons learned from personal experience are of equal importance. Reading about another person's courage inspires courage in all of us.

Autobiographical and Inspirational Books

People who write from personal experience add a dimension that typically does not exist in a purely informational book. The lessons they have learned often provide rare insight. The following books offer a sampling of the various perspectives of people who "have been there" and the coping tools they used.

Anderson, Greg. *The Cancer Conquerer.* New York: Plume/Penguin, 1991.

Anderson, Greg. *50 Essential Things to Do When the Doctor Says It's Cancer.* New York: Plume/Penguin, 1993.

Bloch, Richard, and Annette Bloch. *Fighting Cancer.* Kansas City: Cancer Connection, Inc., 1985.

Bloch, Richard, and Annette Bloch. *Cancer. . . There's Hope.* Kansas City: Cancer Connection, Inc., 1985.

Blumberg, Rena. *Headstrong: A Story of Conquests and Celebrations.* New York: Crown. 1982.

Brady, Judy, ed. *1 in 3: Women with Cancer Confront an Epidemic.* Pittsburgh: Cleis Press, 1991.

Frank, Arthur. *At the Will of the Body: Reflections on Illness.* Boston: Houghton Mifflin, 1991.

Graham, Jory. *In the Company of Others*: *Understanding the Human Needs of Cancer Patients*. New York: Harcourt Brace Jovanovich, 1982.

Gunther, John. *Death Be Not Proud*. New York: Harper & Row, 1949.

Harper, T. and R. Harper. *I Choose to Fight*. Englewood Cliffs, NJ: Prentice Hall, 1984.

Harpham, Wendy Schlessel. *Diagnosis: Cancer: Your Guide Through the First Few Months*. New York: W. W. Norton, 1992.

Ireland, Jill. *Life Wish*. New York: Little, Brown & Co., 1988.

Kahane, Deborah. *No Less A Woman: Ten Women Shatter the Myths about Breast Cancer*. New York: Prentice Hall, 1990. (An educational and inspirational account of ten women written by a breast cancer survivor and educator.)

Kaye, Ronnie. *Spinning Straw Into Gold*. New York: Fireside/Simon & Schuster, 1991.

Kelly, Orville E. *Until Tomorrow Comes*. New York: Everest House, 1979.

Mullan, Fitzhugh. *Vital Signs: A Young Doctor's Struggle with Cancer*. New York: Farrar, Straus & Giroux, 1983.

Murcia, Andy. *Man to Man: When the Woman You Love has Breast Cancer*. New York: St. Martin's Press, 1989. (Written by Ann Jillian's husband and another man married to a woman with breast cancer.)

Pepper, C.B. *We the Victors*. New York: New American Library, 1985. (Stories of several people who survived cancer and how they did it.)

Photopulos, Georgia. *Of Tears and Triumph*. New York: Cogden & Weed, 1988.

Radner, Gilda. *It's Always Something*. New York: Simon & Shuster, 1989. (Comedienne Gilda Radner's struggle with ovarian cancer.)

Ryan, Cornelius, and Kathryn Morgan Ryan. *A Private Battle*. New York: Simon & Shuster, 1979. (Kathryn Ryan's compilation of journals she discovered after Cornelius Ryan's death from prostate cancer.)

Sarton, May. *Recovering: A Journal*. New York: W.W. Norton, 1986. (A personal journal putting recovery from mastectomy into the context of everyday life.)

Soiffer, Bill. *Life in the Shadow: Living with Cancer*. San Francisco: Chronicle Books, 1991.

Spingarn, Natalie Davis. *Hanging in There: Living Well on Borrowed Time*. Briarcliff Manor, NY: Stein & Day, 1982.

Tsongas, Paul. *Heading Home*. New York: Knopf, 1984.

Turnage, Anne Shaw. *More than You Dare to Ask: The First Year of Living with Cancer*. 1992. Order c/o Can Care, 11612 Memorial Drive, Houston, TX 77024.

Wadler, Joyce. *My Breast: One Woman's Cancer Story*. Reading, Mass.: Addison-Wesley, 1992. (Short, but insightful account written by a journalist about her own experience.)

Zumwalt, Admiral Elmo Jr. and Lieutenant Elmo III with John Pekkanen. *My Father, My Son*. New York: Macmillan, 1986.

Other Publications

BMT Newsletter
1985 Spruce Avenue
Highland Park, Illinois 60035
(708) 831-1913

Excellent source of information for and about people who have had bone marrow transplants. A book explaining bone marrow transplant is also available from this address.

Coping Magazine
2019 N. Carothers
Franklin, TN 37064
(615) 790-2400

Informative magazine published four or five times a year with articles on living with cancer, advances in treatment and research, and inspirational pieces.

Living Through Cancer
323 Eighth Street SW
Albuquerque, NM 87102
    (505) 242-3263

Personal stories, poetry, book reviews, articles, and resource lists.

NCCS Networker
1010 Wayne Avenue
Silver Spring, MD 20910
(301) 650-8868

Newsletter of the National Coalition for Cancer Survivorship

Surviving!
Stanford University Medical Center
Patient Research Center, Room H0103
Division of Radiation Oncology
300 Pasteur Drive
Stanford, CA 94305
(415) 723-7881

Patient newsletter providing all kinds of information for and about cancer survivors.

Videotapes

The Challenge of Cancer: Myths and Realities

This American Cancer Society (ACS) video gives clear information on specific medical terms relating to cancer and its treatment. An excellent video for people who are just confronting cancer for the first time.

The Cancer Experience: Who Are You Now?

Produced by Cerenex Pharmaceuticals in cooperation with the ACS, this video does a good job of describing emotions, family relationships, and friendships and a look at how people change as they face cancer.

The Significant Journey: Breast Cancer Survivors and the Men who Love Them

This excellent video is produced by the Minnesota Division of the ACS, with a grant from the 3M Foundation. Couples share their insights on maintaining intimate relationships through the breast cancer experience.

The above three videos can be obtained from:
American Cancer Society
1599 Clifton Road NE
Atlanta, GA 30329-4251

Cancer: Its Effect on Self-Image and Intimate Relationships

Provides a candid look at how cancer affects a person's body image, relationships, and sexuality. The importance of intimacy is discussed through the views and experiences of several cancer patients.

Facing Cancer

In a series of interviews, cancer patients describe the emotional and social impact cancer has had on their lives.

The two videos on the preceding page can be obtained from:
Lincoln Medical Education Foundation
Attention: Cancer Video
4600 Valley Road
Lincoln, NE 68510

Fight for Your Life: Survival Techniques for Those With Cancer

This 2 1/2 hour video documents the struggle and eventual survival of four cancer patients. Gives you step-by-step guide to skills needed to fight for life. This video is available from:

Fight for Your Life Company
63 Elm Street
Camden, ME 04843

Voyage to Byzantium

The poet William Butler Yeats wrote of Byzantium, the holy city of the imagination, a symbol of triumph over time and death. This beautifully filmed video follows several cancer survivors as they take a boat ride and discuss the hopeful aspects of their cancer journey. This film is available from:

Memphis Cancer Center Foundation
1068 Cresthaven Suite 500
Memphis, TN 38119

Solitudes: Loon Country by Canoe

A visual wilderness experience with sound of the stroke of a paddle, wind through the trees, cry of the loon, wail of timber wolf. It creates a wilderness refuge for resting the body, mind, and soul. This film is available from:

Moss Music Group, Inc.
200 Varick Street
New York, NY 10014

Many other videos are available through the *Coping Magazine* book/video/audio catalog. To receive a free copy, write or call:

Coping Books
2019 North Carothers
Franklin, TN 37064
(615) 790-2400

The list of possible resources is endless. I CAN COPE facilitators make the search easier for class participants by compiling a reference library before the start of class. That library usually includes many books and pamphlets not listed here, including local resources, as well as videotapes, relaxation tapes, and records. You can check out these materials free of charge when you attend I CAN COPE classes.

Supplying yourself with adequate resources is another way to take charge of your life. If you learn to control everything that is subject to your control, it helps you forget about what is beyond your control.

Suggested Reading

To learn more about topics discussed in Chapter 7, the following reading material is recommended.

Delong, M. *Practical and Legal Concerns of Cancer Patients and Their Families: A Handbook for Caregivers.* Durham, NC: Duke University Medical Center, 1984. Material collected at Duke Comprehensive Cancer Center, designed for all health care professionals who care for people with cancer.

Harrington, Geri. *The Health Insurance Fact and Answer Book.* New York: Harper and Row, 1985. Helps explain group, individual, disability, and indemnity policies. Helpful to most people, including those on Medicare.

Harrington, Geri. *The Medicare Answer Book.* New York: Harper & Row, 1982. Helpful for anyone on Medicare; publisher will send free Medicare update to inform you on major new developments.

Johnson, A.M. *The Ultimate Organizer.* New York: Ballantine Books, 1984. Tips on organizing one's affairs—very comprehensive.

Larschan, Edward J., and Richard J. Larschan. *The Diagnosis is Cancer.* Palo Alto: Bull Publishing, 1986. Written by a cancer survivor, gives excellent information on hospitalization, money matters, and legal issues.

Mullan, Fitzhugh, and Barbara Hoffman. *Charting the Journey: An Almanac of Practical Resources for Cancer Survivors.* Mount Vernon, NY: Consumer Reports Books, 1990.

Nassif, Janet Zhun. *The Home Health Care Solution.* New York: Harper & Row, 1985. Comprehensive coverage of caring for sick or elderly, including excellent resource guide.

North Carolina Bar Association. *Living Wills: A Declaration of the Desire for a Natural Death.* 1985.

Petterle, Elmo A. *Getting Your Affairs in Order.* Bolinas, CA: Shelter Publications, 1993. Practical guide for making life easier for survivors in the event of death. Very useful.

Personal Inventory of _____ Date _____

Address _____ Birthplace _____ Wife's Maiden Name _____ Birthplace _____

Birthdate _____ SS Number _____ Birthdate _____ SS Number _____

Children
Name _____
Address _____
Name _____
Address _____
Name _____
Address _____

Next of Kin
Name _____
Address _____

Employment
Company Name _____

Address _____

Person Familiar with Company _____
Benefits _____

Personal Papers
Item _____ Location _____

Personal Property
AUTOMOBILES
Make _____ Model _____ Year _____

MAJOR HOUSEHOLD FURNISHINGS
_____
_____

Personal Items
Jewelry, Furs, Personal Effects (Item & Value)
_____
_____

Insurance
LIFE
Company _____ Amount, Policy # _____

HEALTH & ACCIDENT
_____

AUTOMOBILE
_____

HOMEOWNERS
_____

OTHER POLICIES & MEMOS
_____

Stocks & Bonds
Name/No. _____ Quantity _____ Price _____ Date _____

Counselors
Attorney _____

Banker _____
Broker _____
Accountant _____
Insurance Agent _____
Doctors _____

Clergymen _____
Friends & Business Associates _____

Real Estate
Address of Residence _____

City and State _____

Title in Name of _____

Mortgage Held by _____
LOCATION OF REAL ESTATE PAPERS _____

OTHER REAL ESTATE _____

Personal Banking
SAVINGS & CHECKING ACCOUNTS
Institution _____ Account Number _____

SAFE DEPOSIT BOXES
_____

OTHER ACCOUNTS & MEMOS
_____

Funeral Arrangements
Arrangements Have Been Made With _____

Family Burial Plot _____

Special Requests
_____

Request and Donations
Minister _____
Favorite Hymns _____

Scripture Passages _____

Pall Bearers _____

Type of Service _____
Friends & Relatives to be Notified _____

Life Saving Measures desired to prolong life? _____

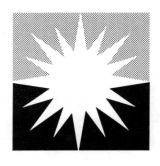

When you have come to the edge

of all the light you know

And are about to step off into

the dark of the unknown,

Faith is knowing one of two

things will happen:

There will be something solid to

stand on

OR

You will be taught to fly.

Author Unknown

CHAPTER EIGHT

CELEBRATING LIFE

The peace that passeth all understanding.

"I kept repeating those words over and over again as I was heading into surgery," recalls Malinda. "I was so afraid. Somehow I felt more secure knowing that maybe I wasn't alone."

After two years of sharing and caring, the friendship between Malinda and Debbie has become a close one. Today they warm themselves by the fire at a December gathering of several I CAN COPE graduates. Lothair, Dick, Bill, and all of their wives are also a part of the group. Over holiday treats and hot buttered rum, they talk about the changes cancer has brought to their lives. They talk about celebrating life.

Malinda is the first to speak. "In order to get myself turned around and able to fight on, I have turned my back on the negative. I simply keep looking until I find something positive. But more than anything, I feel there is something bigger than me out there helping me. Guiding me. And I need that."

Some call it religion. Some call it the power within themselves. Some call it spirituality. Most people agree that a cancer diagnosis represents a spiritual crisis, regardless of your belief system. A confrontation with mortality tends to nudge people into a journey of self-discovery, starting with the question: "What does it all mean, and what is my purpose here?" For some, the journey is easier than for others. Those who find it most difficult tend to become alienated from God, consumed with anger over being chosen as the "cancer victim." Those who weather the crisis well understand that cancer is a physical ailment of a physical body, and they embrace spiritual guidance to help them cope with a physical problem. A strong sense of spirituality can be a lifeline for people learning to live with cancer. The resources offered in the previous chapter are valuable external tools. But for some people, all the external tools are meaningless without internal peace.

Lothair exudes internal peace. Despite the fact that he is weak and cannot socialize for long periods, he was insistent on attending today's gathering. He shares his perception of spirituality with the group. "People sometimes criticize me for my constant positive attitude. Even my son is afraid I'm not facing up to reality— that I'm not admitting how sick I really am. You know what I tell them? I'm not afraid to die. Because I know where I'm going." He smiles and points heavenward. His steel blue eyes radiate inner peace. "But for today, I'm still in the business of living."

Debbie's religion is not so clear-cut. She is not a member of an organized church, but she does believe in some sort of divine intervention. "When I really need something, it happens for me," she says. "I know somebody's pulling the strings to make that happen. I honestly believe there is a reason I had this brain tumor. I think I need a little more guidance to help me understand the reason, though." She laughs and shakes her head to show off a full head of blond hair. "Now tell me God didn't have something to do with this," she continues, pulling at her hair. "The oncologist told me I'd never get it back. I proved him wrong."

Debbie is looking for a reason why she was the one to have the brain tumor. She's trying to make some sense out of the chaos. In Victor Frankl's book *Man's Search for Meaning*, the author postulates that people who find meaning in their lives tend to be stronger survivors. Assigning meaning is a part of the journey of self-discovery. Successful survivors often discover inner resources that fan the flame of hope. Call it what you may—courage, effort, determination, endurance, love, or faith. All are inner resources, and all nurture the will to live.

Unlike Debbie, Dick wasn't so lucky when it comes to hair. "People ask me how cancer has changed my life. I tell them now I wear a hat all the time," he quips. Always ready with a joke, especially on himself, Dick is usually not so quick to volunteer sensitive information about his cancer. What part did spirituality play in his encounter with cancer? "Even though both my wife and I had pretty much fallen away from our religion, I did receive communion when I was in the hospital. Without warning, I found myself crying. I guess it's because I didn't know what I had ahead of me."

"None of us did," Malinda breaks in. "That's why it's easy to have faith in some sort of higher being. Whenever cancer throws me a new curve, God is in there to help soften the blow. How else could I have found a wonderful home like Evie's if God hadn't been helping?"

The challenge of starting at the beginning and rebuilding a life after cancer is a challenge these ten people share with one out of every three Americans. And no two people will go about doing it in exactly the same way.

For Bill, ten years elapsed between his first confrontation with cancer and the surprise recurrence. At five years, doctors were calling him cured. He was even starting to believe it himself. But Bill's indomitable spirit carried him through the second time around equally well. He even telephoned the coauthor of this book from his hospital bed to say, "The weeds are growing back in my lawn. You need to modify your book." Today Bill is again cancer free, twice conquering testicular cancer, a disease that would have killed him not many years earlier. The small company his father helped him start is now thriving. And instead of doing all the work himself, he has hired a manager, so now he spends more time enjoying life. "I try not to make cancer a big part of my life anymore. I need to move ahead without being afraid."

Malinda's future is not so certain. "I've simply accepted the fact that cancer is part of my life," she says. "I'm hooked up most of the time receiving megadoses of 5FU. The goal isn't cure anymore; it's control. My last bone scan showed the tumor to be about the same size. I'm just thankful for every day I have. Especially when I feel this good."

Lothair nods in agreement. "Life isn't always a diamond-studded stairway to the sky," he adds. "And this cancer hasn't exactly been a picnic. But I believe confident prayer is a powerful thing. Today, like Malinda, Ruth and I pray for control of my cancer. The doctors have been successful at getting rid of my pain. That means I'm able to enjoy every day we have together."

Almost 13 years have gone by since most of Dick's right lung was removed. Cancer is not so ever-present in his life, but its lesson lingers on. "I've gone up and looked over the edge. I stared death in the face when I had that surgery. My prognosis was not good. When you come that close to death, it changes your way of thinking."

At the time of diagnosis, none of these people knew what was ahead. Today, they all continue to work at moving forward. John, Hazel, Dick, Bill, Dave, and Debbie are free of cancer—for now. Does that make them survivors? Is a survivor someone who is free of cancer? Not according to Malinda, Lothair, Jim, and Lou, who continue to fight the illness, yet live each day to the fullest. Even though some are free of cancer and some still have it with them every day, they all consider themselves survivors.

Exactly what is a survivor? The American Cancer Society uses the following definition: "From the time of discovery and for the balance of life, an individual diagnosed with cancer is a survivor." Likewise, the National Coalition for Cancer Survivorship says that survivorship begins at the time of diagnosis and continues through and beyond treatment. Survivors include people living with cancer, in a state of remission, and those who are completely free of disease.

Remember that surviving medically doesn't necessarily make a person a survivor. Some people, regardless of the stage or expected outcome of their disease, just tend to get along better from day to day than others. They are thriving, not just surviving. Why? Because they have developed a set of coping skills that allow them to reduce their emotional stress.

Effective Coping Strategies

- Confront the problem directly.

- Look at the situation as a problem to be solved.

- Insist on complete information.

- Expect positive change.

- Be flexible; take things as they come.

- Divide major events into step-by-step tasks.

- Utilize resources.

- Seek support.

What personal lifestyles and habits seem to separate a survivor from a thriving survivor? When cancer becomes a part of your life, what is still within your control? The people in this book, along with cancer survivors around the world, have been able to effect positive change as a result of cancer's initial negative impact. The suggestions that follow have allowed many people to live quality lives despite the fact that uncertainty prevails.

Be Open and Express Your Feelings Honestly

Concentrate on what's best for you. Don't worry about pleasing others. If you feel bad, say so. If you need help, ask for it. Stop hiding your feelings in order to make others feel better. "I think I learned that lesson the hard way," says Malinda. "I was so good at covering up my cancer, my husband didn't really take me seriously. Now I know better. I'm fighting for me. And for my health. Everything else is secondary."

Maybe it's Dave's German heritage that makes it so difficult for him to get in touch with his emotions, and even more difficult for him to express those emotions. Loretta claims it's probably her Italian heritage that causes her to react just the opposite. When the two of them left the doctor's office after learning of Dave's recurrence, Loretta wanted to have coffee and talk. Dave wanted to go back to work.

Their two daughters know their Dad well. His actions show his love for them, but sometimes the words just don't come. One daughter found it easier to express her feelings in writing and sent her father a heartfelt note for Father's Day. She finished by saying: "I feel a strange kind of grief that lives near the surface of my consciousness, ready to leap out at moments like this. I think the reason it lurks is because I feel I could lose you at any time and not have said how I felt. That would be too painful to bear. I guess it's the German in us that makes us bottle up our true feelings inside, and it takes one hell of a lot for us to let them out and truly express what we are feeling. I love you, Dad. It's plain and simple, that's how it is. You've helped to shape me into the person that I am and I thank you for that."

It would be a tragedy to leave beautiful words such as these unsaid. Take time today to openly and honestly express your feelings to those who are important to you.

Guard Against Depression

Mood swings are normal. Particularly right after the diagnosis, it is common to feel disoriented and confused because of depression. But unchecked depression is both emotionally and physically draining. Research is starting to recognize the connection between attitude and the immune system. Guarding against depression may be one of the most powerful inner controls you have over the course of your illness.

Instead of regarding cancer as a burden, think of it as a problem to be solved. Then become the problem solver. List the things within your control. Then develop a plan of action for controlling them.

When depression strikes, and it undoubtedly will, view it as a cloudburst, a brief rainstorm that will soon pass. Use one of the coping strategies in this chapter as a temporary shelter to protect you from the storm. Take care of yourself by indulging in a favorite activity. Go out of your way to help someone. Gain strength from your faith. Seek support from friends, loved ones, or a support network. Watch a good movie and have a good laugh.

The trick is to do what you can to not get down and stay down. Feel free to call on others to help you do it. "When I feel like having a pity party," says Malinda, "I call Debbie and we pig out on junk food. It's probably not good for us physically. But it's fun, and it gets me out of my depression."

Refuse to be Limited

In the book *Getting Well Again*, the authors point out that people with cancer are capable of far more physical activity than they would believe possible. And people who engage in a regular exercise program tend to develop a healthier psychological profile. It may seem easier to not get dressed. You may have convinced yourself you're too sick to get out of bed. People are coaxing you to "save your strength." But by limiting yourself physically, you are also limiting yourself mentally. Your best route to staying healthy with cancer is to keep both mind and body active.

"Get out and do something," is Bill's advice to anyone feeling burdened by cancer or its treatment. Motion is sacred. Getting out and involved in some type of active physical program not only enhances overall health, but helps aid regularity and prevents insomnia.

Seek Support from Others

The success of people who have attended I CAN COPE has proved the life-enhancing value of emotional support given by others. Cancer patients truly have a bond that surpasses a healthy person's understanding. Thriving survivors use that bond to build themselves back up emotionally as well as physically. They can then reenter the world as slightly changed, but stronger, individuals.

"Where would we be without each other?" is a question these group members often ask one another. For John and Hazel, it has been 15 years since they first registered for I CAN COPE classes. Today former support group members remain close friends. "Because of attending the group, our knowledge of cancer has come a long way. And every year, new people in the group inspired us all over again with their courage and hope. But the most rewarding part is that we have helped others along the way."

Withdrawing from social contacts can lead to depression. Getting out and seeking new acquaintances is a hedge against depression. "And don't forget," adds John, "this group is good for a lot of laughs, too."

Identify Something to Live For

Jim and Shirley were devastated when they learned Jim's cancer had metastasized to his liver. But they were committed to living life despite the limited success of his chemotherapy. They made plans for an extended winter vacation in Florida. They identified something to live for. And early in December they went.

Shirley's first letter started out, "When we saw the sign 'Caution: Adults Having Fun,' we knew we were at the right place." They were referred to an oncologist nearby, and Jim continued to receive his cancer care while basking in Florida's sunshine.

Bill has always loved machines, especially cars. He's looking forward to enjoying the cars of the future. "I've been driving for 20 years, and I'm constantly being surprised by the new things they come up with. I can't wait to see what future technology brings. I'm waiting for the discovery of alternative fuels that are cost effective." And Bill has a four-year-old nephew. "I intend to watch that kid grow up. I want him to remember me."

Having something to live for makes life just that much more valuable. You may be living for a spouse; to see your children graduate; to retire and travel a little. Whatever the goal, keep it alive. It will help keep you alive.

Get Rid of Excess Baggage

What are you carrying around that is weighing you down? We all carry excess baggage because we find change difficult. We weigh more than we should because dieting is difficult. We hold onto our jobs because finding another one is difficult. The old saying "When God closes a door, he opens a window," may pertain to you. Perhaps the time has come to reassess your life. Are your loved ones being supportive? Is your job fulfilling? Are you pursuing outside interests that are healthy? Do you have a spiritual relationship?

Confront your problems. Don't ignore them. Although confrontation is difficult in the short term, the long-term impact of any positive change you make will provide for a happier, healthier future.

Have Goals—Make Plans

Thriving survivors learn to accept cancer's uncertainty as a challenge. They redefine the meaning of the word "future." Dealing with cancer and its treatment may cause you to put plans on hold or force some goals into the background. But don't give up on those goals or totally cancel those plans. They are your link to life.

"Once you've had cancer, you have to accept the fact that your life is going to be different," says Dick. "Today, even though I'm considered cured, I'm sure my long-term goals aren't what they would be if I hadn't had the cancer." Faced with uncertainty, Dick demands the best for himself, both in his job and in his home life. "If I'm unhappy in my job, I find another one. I take a vacation as soon as I've earned it instead of saving up for retirement."

Malinda knows that planning for retirement is unrealistic. "But that doesn't mean I don't have goals," she emphasizes. "I've been putting away money to make a trip to Japan with some artist friends. I've always been interested in Oriental sculpture. I think you have to make plans for the future, no matter how uncertain that future may be."

Take Care of Yourself

Many people still make the mistake of believing taking care of other people is more important than taking care of themselves. Nothing could be further from the truth. When your own tank is on empty, you can't generate enough power to help someone else. Take care of your own needs first; then worry about the needs of others. Make a list of the activities that give you pleasure. Today, and every day from now on, take time to pamper yourself by indulging in at least one of those activities. Taking care of yourself also means eating properly, exercising appropriately, and allowing for quiet time each day to renew your spirit.

Live for This Day

"We are all, it seems, saving ourselves for the senior prom. But many of us forget that somewhere along the way we must learn to dance." Author Alan Harrington made these comments regarding retirement. But his words ring true for most of us as we go about our daily routine. We hurry to get it all done, without stopping to consider what we are doing. Or why.

Elisabeth Kubler-Ross, who has written extensively on the topic of death and dying, says, "When you finally understand that each day you awaken could be the last day you have, you take the time that day to grow, to become more of who you really are, to reach out to other human beings."

"This year as Evie and I put the decorations on the tree," says Malinda, "I chose each spot carefully. I looked at every decoration and made her tell me its history. Just think about it. If you knew you would never see your Christmas decorations again, wouldn't you spend more time enjoying them?"

We all want to believe we're living for the day, hugging our loved ones, stopping to smell the roses. But are we? Unless we consciously think about it, first in the morning as we plan our day, and then periodically throughout the day, we often lose sight of this goal.

Face and Accept Your Own Mortality

When cancer is diagnosed, people often experience a two-part loss. They not only lose their good health. They also lose their sense of immortality and are forced to begin accepting the fact that death—their death—is part of life. Getting to the point where you are able to accept your own mortality takes time and effort. It's often a slow and painful process. But those who have succeeded will tell you it's worth the effort. The new awareness of life's precious quality heightens and sharpens every experience.

John A. MacDonald, in his book *Living with Cancer*, talks about achieving his own acceptance after a lung cancer diagnosis. "My appreciation of life increased. The warmth of each kiss, the tenderness of each caress, the sound of laughter were enhanced. There was a heightened awareness of each sunny day, of the beauty of flowers, of the singing of a bird. One soon realizes how precious life is when it appears certain that it will be curtailed."

Lothair often talks of the inevitability of death. Perhaps he's lucky, he claims, because he has been given fair warning of what lies ahead. "Death is certain for all of us," he says. "How we live out our remaining days, however many they may be, is up to us."

Putting life and death into perspective is an immense challenge. Life is undeniably a terminal illness, but people facing cancer come face to face with this reality sooner rather than later. Inevitably, all must make peace with their own mortality before they can thrive.

Remember That Being Afraid is Normal

Fear is part of this disease. Some days you are able to go forward without letting negative thoughts get in your way. Other days you are paralyzed with fear. Will the cancer recur? Will I be in pain? Has it spread? "I'd like to say you put it behind you and never think about it," says John, who has been free of cancer for almost 11 years. "But I can't. Every time I'm due for a checkup, it all comes back. Thankfully, after I get a good report, I can get back to living a normal life again."

Facts negate fear. Many times, the imagined fears turn out to be far worse than reality. Getting adequate information in a timely fashion will help diminish fears. Don't wait and wonder if you think you have new symptoms. Check them out and put your mind at rest. Expect fears to recur, but don't dwell on them.

Gain Strength from Your Faith

Theologian Paul Tillich said, "Faith means being grasped by a power that is greater than we are, a power that shakes us and turns us and transforms us and heals us. Surrender to this power is faith."

Those who are lucky enough to have a strong faith find immense comfort in prayer. Lothair, whose greatest fear was pain, believes his prayers were answered. "I'm not suffering, and that was what I feared most. Ask and you shall receive. It has always worked for me."

Malinda remembers reading the Biblical book of Job when she got home from the hospital. "I thought of all his trials and the things he had to go through, and yet he kept holding on. It's funny how certain things pull you through, and you don't know exactly why."

Giving in to something higher than yourself can provide great comfort in times of stress. You realize that you don't have to do it alone, that you can trust in something to help you. Even if your own faith is limited, be willing to accept the prayers and support of family and friends. The faith and hope they channel toward your recovery can be very meaningful.

Nourish Hope

Nothing is inevitable, so starting today, reject all notions of inevitability. Richard Bloch faced a serious lung cancer, fought it, and won. He says: "There is no type of cancer for which there is no treatment; and there is no type of cancer from which some people have not been cured."

Hope may be your most powerful ally in the struggle to find balance in your life. Without hope, the cancer can become your fate. Instead of having cancer, it has you. With hope, you can realistically accept your situation, but also see its redeeming aspects. Guard against thoughts of becoming a statistic. You are a person with cancer. At the time of diagnosis, no one knows where you will fit in the statistical model. As Malinda told her doctor, "If 3 percent of the people with this type of cancer are cured, I want to be part of that 3 percent." Learn to believe in miracles. Then picture yourself as part of one.

Cultivate a Positive, Optimistic Attitude

Look past the bad to find the good. Believe you have the resources within you to confront this challenge—because you do. A positive attitude doesn't mean you're smiling all the time. It's normal to be depressed and cry. Someone with the right attitude accepts those sad times, works through them, and moves on. Losing yourself to depression and pessimism is not only physically and emotionally draining, but it's also a big time waster. Hold your head high, keep up your physical appearance and maintain an attitude of cheerfulness.

Laughter can be the best medicine when your mood is low. Seek out a friend who makes you laugh. Read the newspaper comics from cover to cover each day. Lose yourself in a humorous movie or video. Make a joke on yourself. The theoretical link between attitude and the immune system is too important to ignore. Although no one can predict at the outset what your survival chances might be, a person's mental attitude and adaptation to the cancer can affect both the quantity and quality of your life.

Find Purpose for Your Existence

German philosopher, poet, and critic Friedrich Nietzsche said, "He who has a why to live can bear almost any how." Victor Frankl discovered that those who find meaning in their lives are the strongest survivors. Each of us has a unique gift. Each of us is on earth for a reason. Most of us never stop to figure out what that reason is. Cancer's wakeup call jolts the thriving survivor out of complacency and into action. Forced to look deep inside, most people can discover the niche where they fit and can define their purpose, the way they want to live. Taking steps to fulfill that purpose and being committed to your ideals can be richly rewarding. It gives you some control over your life and answers the question "Why am I here?"

Many discover that in giving, they receive, and in loving, they truly experience love. They find purpose in reaching out to help others. Committed volunteers are the backbone of the American Cancer Society. They provide a lifeline for newly diagnosed cancer patients. Fitzhugh Mullan, a physician and cancer survivor, was instrumental in getting the National Coalition of Cancer Survivors off the ground. He then became active in lobbying for health care reform that benefits people with cancer. Richard Bloch, another cancer survivor, formed the R.A. Bloch Foundation, which provides information and support to thousands of people every year. After his recovery from lung cancer, Greg Anderson, author and founder of the The Cancer Conqueror's Foundation, committed his life to teaching patients and their families how to cope with cancer.

Each of us has a purpose. If you're having difficulty identifying that purpose, think back in your life to the times that were most stimulating. Think back to an activity that has always given you satisfaction. Think back to a day or a time when you truly believed you were in the right place at the right time, achieving what you were meant to achieve, and your efforts made a difference. What were you doing? Do you look forward to doing it again? Perhaps that's a first step in identifying your purpose. Thriving survivors are committed to the standards, the values, and the lifestyle defined by this purpose. Meaningful activity keeps them alive.

Live a Life of High Quality

Maybe it's time to get off the express train and start enjoying the countryside. There's nothing like a life-threatening illness to force a total reassessment of your values. Are you living your life according to your values or according to society's values?

Before his bout with testicular cancer, Bill tested life to its limits. Three-wheel vehicles. Motorcycles. Snowmobiles. Fast cars. "My motto used to be, 'Live fast, die young, and leave a good-looking corpse," he recalls. "Now I have a little more respect for life. Every day that comes is a blessing. I don't take that lightly." Bill still has his toys. But they aren't quite as crazy. He's constantly trading cars, his most recent acquisition being a Corvette for his wife. But he's not driving so fast anymore. "Now I have radio-controlled cars. I can race them without hurting myself."

A life of high quality is filled with peaks and valleys. Hearing the words, "You have cancer," represented a deep valley for the ten people in this book. But they survived the shock of those words, recognized the cancer as a problem to be solved, and then devised a plan for moving forward with their lives. They pulled themselves out of the valley and became acutely aware of the peak moments they could still enjoy, cancer or no cancer.

What is a peak moment? It's that precious time when you know life just can't get any better. Your peak moment may be watching a sunset, a time when you stand quietly in awe of nature. It may be watching your baby's birth and then celebrating every "first" that child achieves—the first step, the first word, and the first long climb up school bus steps.

Peak moments often occur in relationships, times when you feel truly connected to another individual, or when the spirit of human kindness overwhelms you. Finally, peak moments occur when people spiritually connect with a power larger than themselves. Peak moments elicit strong human reactions—special feelings of awe, tenderness, wonder, humility, pride, or simply a profound thankfulness for being alive today. Thriving survivors are tuned in to peak moments and celebrate each one as it comes along.

Paul Tsongas, former U.S. Senator from Massachusetts, was forced to reassess the quality of his life after a diagnosis of lymphoma. At the age of 42, with three young children, this rising politician gave up his powerful position to renew and revitalize his relationship with his family. In his book *Heading Home*, Tsongas says, "The lymphoma caused me to realize the preciousness of the moments of a child's development. I would have spent too much time away from my daughters had I continued my career. Life is a search for balance. We all have to bring the scales back to center."

Balance. Bringing the scales back to center. That's what staying healthy with cancer is all about. And the best way to achieve that balance is to concentrate on living a life of high quality each and every day. Choose your priorities carefully. Dwell on the positive aspects of the present. The future will take care of itself.

And what of the future? Dr. Lewis Thomas, former head of the Memorial Sloan-Kettering Cancer Center, often talks about the future of knowledge. He once said, "We have hardly begun to learn. We have not come to the end of knowledge by a long shot; we have only come to the edge of it."

At the National Cancer Institute, Steven Rosenberg continues to make strides toward that end of knowledge as it relates to understanding the mystery of cancer. A child at the end of World War II, Dr. Rosenberg witnessed the pain his family experienced after living through the horrors of the Holocaust. Because of this, he identified his purpose at a young age. He knew before age 10 that he wanted to "find things that no one else knew." He had an obsession with doing something that would alleviate suffering. His indefatigable and continuous efforts to fine-tune his brain child—adoptive immunotherapy—to accomplish that goal are taking science closer and closer to the elusive cure for cancer.

Only at the edge of knowledge? It's an uplifting thought. The decades ahead should hold great promise for cancer research. No one can predict what is around the corner for the individual diagnosed with cancer today. But there is certainly reason for hope.

Suggested Reading

To learn more about topics discussed in Chapter 8, the following reading material is recommended.

Benjamin, H.H. *From Victim to Victor: The Wellness Community Guide to Fighting for Recovery*. Los Angeles: Jeremy P. Tarcher, Inc., 1987. Philosophical approach to fighting cancer as viewed by the Wellness Community.

Glassman, Judith. *The Cancer Survivors—And How They Did It*. New York: Dial Press, 1983. Inner and outer resources people have used.

Morra, Marion and Eve Potts. Triumph: *Getting Back to Normal When You Have Cancer.* New York: Avon Books, 1990.

Nessin, Susan and Judith Ellis. *Cancervive: The Challenge of Life after Cancer*. Boston: Houghton-Mifflin, 1991.

Pitzele, Sefra Kobrin. *We Are Not Alone: Learning to Live with Chronic Illness*. Minneapolis: Thompson & Company, Inc. 1985.

Williams, Wendy. *The Power Within: True Stories of Exceptional Patients Who Fought Back with Hope*. New York: Harper & Row. 1990.

If you need more comprehensive information about cancer, the following medical textbooks might be helpful.

Medical Texts

Abeloff, M.D. (ed). *Complications of Cancer: Diagnosis and Management*. Baltimore: The Johns Hopkins University Press, 1979.

Chabner, Bruce A. et al, (eds). *Cancer Chemotherapy: Principles and Practice*. Philadelphia: Lippincott, 1990.

DeVita, Vincent T., Jr.; Hellman, S.; and Rosenberg, S.A. (eds). *Cancer: Principles and Practices of Oncology*. 3rd edition. Philadelphia: Lippincott Company, 1990.

Fischer, David S. and M. Tish Knopf (eds). *Cancer Chemotherapy Handbook: Treatment and Care*, 3rd edition, Chicago: Year Book Medical Publishers, 1990.

Groenwald, Susan L. et al (eds). *Cancer Nursing: Principles and Practice*. Jones and Bartlett, 1993.

Haskell, Charles M. (ed). *Cancer Treatment*. New York: W.B. Saunders, 1990.

Holland, Jimmie C., and Julia Rowland (eds). *Handbook of Psychooncology: Psychological Care of the Patient with Cancer*. New York: Oxford University Press, 1989.

Howland, W.S., and G.C. Carlton. *Critical Care of the Cancer Patient*. Chicago: Year Book Medical Publishers, 1985.

Johnson, B.L., and J. Gross. *Handbook of Oncology Nursing*. New York: John Wiley, 1985.

Laszlo, John. *Physician's Guide to Cancer Care Complications*. New York: Marcel Dekker, Inc., 1986.

Levy, S.M. *Behavior and Cancer*. San Francisco: Jossey-Bass Publishers, 1985.

Lippman, Marc E., M.D. et al (eds). *Diagnosis and Management of Breast Cancer*. New York: W.B. Saunders, 1988.

Oldham, Robert K. (ed). *Principles of Cancer Biotherapy.* New York: Raven Press, 1987.

Perry, M.C., and Y.W. Yarbrow (eds). *Toxicity of Chemotherapy.* Orlando, FL: Grune & Stratton, Inc., 1984.

Rosenberg, Steven A. and John M. Barry. *The Transformed Cell: Unlocking the Mysteries of Cancer.* New York: G.P. Putnam & Sons, 1992.

Wiernik, P.H. (ed). *Supportive Care of the Cancer Patient.* Mount Kisco, NY: Futura Publishing Company, Inc., 1983.

Wittes, Robert E. (ed). *Manual of Oncologic Therapeutics 1989/1990.* Philadelphia: Lippincott, 1990.

GLOSSARY

Acupressure Using finger pressure on specific body points (the same points used in acupuncture) to treat disease symptoms.

Acute Occurring suddenly or over a short period of time.

Adenocarcinoma Cancer that starts in glandular tissue (such as breast, lung, thyroid, colon, and pancreas).

Adjuvant chemotherapy Using chemotherapy (anti-cancer drugs) in combination with radiation and/or surgery in hopes of preventing or delaying recurrence. It is usually given after all visible signs of cancer have been removed, but there is still a risk that hidden cancer cells remain.

Allogeneic transplant Transferring tissue, usually bone marrow, from one individual to another. Most successful when tissue types match.

Alopecia Partial or complete hair loss, a common side effect of some chemotherapeutic agents or from radiation to the brain.

Alpha-fetoprotein (AFP) A protein that is elevated in the blood of patients with certain forms of cancer, such as liver or testis.

Aneuploid Tumor cells that do not have 46 chromosomes, the normal number in a human cell. Aneuploid tumors tend to have a poorer prognosis.

Antibody A protein made by the body's immune system to neutralize harmful foreign substances (antigens) such as bacteria, viruses, or cancer.

Anticipatory nausea and vomiting A conditioned response where cues that remind the patient of chemotherapy set off the identical physical response created by chemotherapy treatment.

Antidepressant Drug Medication given to relieve feelings of despair or hopelessness.

Antiemetic Medication used to reduce or prevent nausea and vomiting.

Antigen Any substance causing the body to activate the immune system and produce antibodies.

Aspiration Removal of fluid or tissue with a hollow needle or tube.

Astrocytoma A brain tumor that can be benign or malignant, accounting for 10% of all brain tumors.

Benign A tumor or tissue that is not malignant (cancerous).

Biological Response Modifiers (BRM) Any agent that boosts the body's immune system by stimulating it, modifying it, or restoring it.

Biopsy Removal of tissue from the body for microscopic examination to determine if cancer cells are present.

Blood Count Measurement test to determine the number of red cells, white cells, and platelets in a blood sample.

Bone Marrow The spongy inner core of the bone that produces blood cells.

Bone Scan An image of the bones taken after injecting radioactive dye to help determine if cancer has spread to the bones.

Brachytherapy Treatment with radioactive material placed in a body cavity.

Cachexia Wasting away of the body often caused by advanced cancer.

Carcinogen An agent that initiates or promotes the development of cancer.

Carcinoma Cancer that originates in the epithelial tissue. Most cancers are carcinomas (80 to 90%).

Catheter A flexible tube inserted in the body to drain fluids or to deliver fluids such as chemotherapy.

CAT Scan or CT Scan A computerized X-ray system that delivers very detailed pictures.

Chemotherapy The treatment of cancer (or other diseases) with drugs.

Clinical Trials Studies in humans of new cancer drugs, initiated after studies with animals.

Colony-Stimulating Factor (CSF) An agent that stimulates the production of disease-fighting cells in the bone marrow, enabling the patient to better tolerate chemotherapy.

Cytology Scientific study of the appearance of cells to determine their origin, structure and functions.

Debulking A procedure that reduces the size of a tumor so further treatment can be performed.

DNA Deoxyribonucleic acid, the type of nucleic acid that carries genetic information.

Durable Power of Attorney A legal document allowing someone else to manage your affairs for you. Unlike a standard power of attorney, it continues if you become permanently incapacitated. In some states, can be used for health care decisions.

Edema Abnormal accumulation of fluid that causes swelling in tissues of the body.

Endoscope A flexible scope used to view the inside of an organ or body cavity.

Estrogen Receptor Test A test done during biopsy of cancerous breast tissue to determine if its growth is dependent on the hormone estrogen.

Flow Cytometry A procedure that measures the amount of DNA in cells, and subsequently helps determine the aggressiveness of the tumor cells.

Gamma Knife A costly device used when stereotactic radiosurgery is performed.

Gene The biologic unit of heredity.

Gene Therapy The use of genes in the treatment of cancer, or other diseases.

Grading A way of describing cancer cells in terms of how malignant or aggressive they are.

Hormonal Therapy Treating cancer by using natural or synthetic hormones to manipulate hormone levels in the body, often causing a tumor to stabilize or shrink.

Hospice A program of caring for patients who are terminally ill with a focus on improving quality of life.

Immune System The body mechanism that fights disease by recognizing and neutralizing foreign cells.

Imagery Essentially the same as visualization, a mind exercise where a person creates a mental picture, like a daydream; used to reduce stress, control pain and fight cancer.

Immunotherapy Therapy that stimulates the body's own defense mechanisms to control cancer or kill cancer cells.

In Situ Cancer in its earliest stage, confined to the place or site where it started.

Infusion Pump A small battery-driven device used to deliver a constant or intermittent flow of anticancer drugs or pain medication.

Interferons Potent natural proteins produced by body's lymphocytes as a "front line" defense against viral infections; used in immunotherapy.

Interleukin A group of natural, hormone-like substances produced in the body that stimulate the growth of specific types of lymphocytes; responsible for helping the immune system fight cancer.

Intravenous (IV) Into a vein.

Laser Therapy Use of an extremely narrow, intense, and controlled light beam to treat cancer.

Leukemia Any of a series of malignant diseases of the blood-forming system.

Living Will A signed document that describes under what conditions a person wants life-sustaining equipment to be used.

Lymph Nodes Small, bean-shaped structures in the body that act as filters, collecting bacteria and cancer cells that are to be processed by the immune system. Nodal involvement means cancer has spread from the primary tumor site to nearby nodes.

Lymphedema Swelling of an arm or leg as a result of damage to lymphatic vessels that connect to lymph nodes; caused by surgery or radiation.

Lymphocytes White blood cells that are responsible for a variety of immune reactions.

Lymphoma A tumor originating in lymphatic tissue (neck, groin, armpit).

Malignant Cancerous, as opposed to benign.

Mammography An X-ray procedure used in the screening and diagnosis of breast cancer.

Mastectomy Surgical removal of the breast, usually as treatment for breast cancer.

Melanoma A highly malignant form of cancer of the skin.

Metastasis Migration of cancer cells from the primary tumor site to other parts of the body by way of the blood stream or lymphatic system, thereby producing cancer spread.

Monoclonal Antibodies A highly specific antibody that can be made in a laboratory; because it can find and attach to specific proteins on cancer cells, research continues on ways to deliver drugs exclusively to tumor cells using these antibodies.

MRI (Magnetic Resonance Imaging) Creates body images using a magnetic field and radio waves, rather than X-ray; produces images similar to a CT scan, but with much greater definition.

Myeloma A cancer of the plasma cells in the bone marrow.

Myelosuppression A decrease in the ability of bone marrow cells to produce blood cells, including white cells, red cells, and platelets.

Neoadjuvant Therapy Therapy given before the primary treatment (surgery) to shrink the cancerous tumor.

Nerve Block A technique using anesthesia to temporarily or permanently relieve pain in a specific area

Nuclear Scan A diagnostic procedure using a radioactive substance to examine different organs in the body

Occult Blood Stool Test Examination of the stool for traces of blood not visible to the naked eye.

Oncogene A defective hereditary unit that controls the development of inherited characteristics and is transmitted on the chromosome. When activated, the oncogene can transform some normal cells into malignant cells.

Oncologist A physician who specializes in cancer. Oncology is the study of tumors, especially cancerous ones.

Ostomy Surgical creation of an artificial opening (stoma) through the abdominal wall for elimination of body waste.

Pathologist A physician who specializes in studying the effects of disease on body tissue.

PET Scan (Positron Emission Tomography) A scan that measures emissions from a radioactive isotope injected in the blood. The scan pinpoints changes in metabolic activity indicative of certain abnormalities.

Platelets Cells in the blood that help it to clot.

Primary Tumor The site where the tumor first appeared.

Progesterone Receptor Test A test done during the biopsy of cancerous breast tissue to determine if the tumor is dependent on the hormone progesterone.

Prognosis The expected or probable outcome of an illness or disease.

PSA Test (Prostate specific antigen) Analysis of blood for levels of a protein produced by the prostate. Elevated level may be an indication of prostate cancer.

Prosthesis An artificial replacement for a missing body part.

Protocols The guidelines that specify how a clinical trial will be conducted.

Proto-oncogenes DNA sequences present in normal cells that are related to oncogenes found in viruses.

Psychoneuroimmunology (PNI) The study of the interrelationships among stress, the emotions, the central nervous system, and the immune system.

Questionable Treatment Methods Treatment that has not undergone testing to determine benefits and risks, thus falling outside the bounds of "mainstream" medicine.

Radiation Therapy The treatment of cancer with high-energy X-rays.

Radon A naturally occurring radioactive gas that comes from uranium and rock and is known to be a cause of cancer.

Recurrence The return of cancer after its apparently complete disappearance.

Remission The decrease or disappearance of all measurable evidence of disease, usually after treatment.

Sarcoma Any malignant tumor arising in the bone, cartilage, fibrous tissue, or muscle.

Scan A view or image of the body's internal organs such as liver, brain, and bone; shows abnormalities in structure or function and helps detect cancer or metastases.

Serotonin A naturally occurring chemical neurotransmitter that plays a part in inhibiting pain in the gastrointestinal tract and has also been implicated in some of the unpleasant side effects of chemotherapy.

Side Effect A secondary, unintentional and usually undesirable effect from a drug or other treatment, in addition to the primary, therapeutic effect.

S-Phase Fraction (SPF) The percentage of cancer cells that are in a specific stage (the synthesis phase) of division in the cell cycle. A high SPF number means that the cells are dividing rapidly and that the tumor is fast growing.

Staging A systematic classification of the extent of spread of tumor to help determine prognosis and treatment.

Standard Treatment Treatment that is currently being used by doctors and has been proven effective in scientific studies.

Stem Cell Generate all blood cells arising in the bone marrow, including red blood cells, white blood cells, and platelets.

Stool Blood Test (See occult blood stool test)

Stress A physical or emotional factor that causes tension in the mind and/or body.

Taxol An anticancer drug derived from the Pacific yew tree that has been primarily used in the treatment of ovarian cancer.

T Cell One of the two major types of lymphocytes (white blood cells) that are part of the body's immune system.

Terminal In cancer, characterizes a person with progressive advanced disease with very limited life expectancy.

Testosterone The most powerful of the male sex hormones.

Tumor An abnormal mass of tissue; may be benign or malignant.

Tumor Board A group of specialists who help doctors prescribe treatment in unusual cases.

Tumor Necrosis Factors (TNF) A naturally produced substance in the body as part of the immune system with the ability to kill cancer cells.

Ultrasound A way to locate and measure solid tumors using very high frequency sound waves.

Undifferentiated Cells Cells that lack specialization in function and structure; the more undifferentiated (abnormal) the cells appear under the microscope, the more malignant the cells are.

Venous Access Device (VAD) A soft, plastic catheter designed to remain in place for indefinite periods while a person receives frequent intravenous fluids during treatment for cancer.

Zofran (Ondansetron) An antiemetic drug that works to reduce episodes of nausea and vomiting following administration of some anti-cancer drugs.

Bibliography

Altman, Roberta and Michael J. Sarg, M.D.: *The Cancer Dictionary*. New York: Facts on File, 1992.

Bell, Loran, R.N., and Eudora Seyfer: *Gentle Yoga: A Guide to Gentle Exercise*. Berkeley, CA: Celestial Arts, 1987.

Benjamin, H.H.: *From Victim to Victor: The Wellness Community Guide to Fighting for Recovery*. Los Angeles: Jeremy P. Tarcher, Inc., 1987.

Benson, Herbert, and Miriam Z. Klipper: *The Relaxation Response*. New York: Avon, 1976.

Boin, Cindy Lampner: *"Should You Participate in a Clinical Trial?"* COPING, January 1991, pp. 48-49.

Bombeck, Erma: *I Want to Grow Hair. I Want to Grow Up. I Want to Go to Boise: Children Surviving Cancer*. New York, NY, Harper Collins, 1989.

Bray, Judith: *O.T.R. Activities of Daily Living* (adapted from "Rehabilitation of Chronic Illness" chapter of *Mind and Body: A Rehabilitation Guide for Cancer Patients and Their Families* by Ernest H. Rosenbaum, M.D., and Isadora R. Rosenbaum.

Brody, Jane E.: *You Can Fight Cancer and Win*. New York: Quadrangle, The New York Times Book Co., 1977.

Bruning, Nancy: *Coping With Chemotherapy: How to Take Care of Yourself While Chemotherapy Takes Care of Your Cancer*. New York: Ballantine Books (Random House), 1993.

Cancer Sourcebook for Nurses, Sixth Edition, 1991.

Cancer Statistics 1993, CA-A Cancer Journal for Clinicians, American Cancer Society, January/February 1993, Vol. 43, No. 1

1993 Cancer Facts and Figures. New York: American Cancer Society, 1993.

Cantor, Robert Chernin: *And A Time To Live*. New York: Harper & Row, 1978.

Carter, B.: *"Cancer Survivorship: A Topic For Nursing Research,"* Oncology Nursing Forum, Vol. 16, No. 3, 1989, pp. 435-437.

Chemotherapy and You: A Guide to Self Help During Treatment. Bethesda, Maryland: Office of Cancer Communication, National Cancer Institute, 1990.

Clark, Gary M. and William L. McGuire, M.D. "New Biologic Prognostic Factors in Breast Cancer," *Oncology*, May 1989, pp. 49-54.

Clark, Matt with Mary Hager, Mariana Gosnell, Nancy Stadtman and Daniel Shapiro: "Search for a Cure," *Newsweek,* Dec. 16, 1985, pp. 60-65.

Cohn, Victor: "Releasing the Power of Hope," *The Washington Post/Health*, June 2, 1992, p.10.

"Colony-Stimulating Factors—Helping Blood Cells Grow." *BMT Newsletter, November,* 1992.

Coping With Cancer. Bethesda, Maryland: Office of Cancer Communications, National Cancer Institute, 1980.

Costello, Alice M., R.N.: "Supporting the Patient with Problems Related to Body Image," (from American Cancer Society Professional Education Publication entitled *Emotional Problems of Patients with Cancer; Nursing Intervention).*

Cousins, Norman.: "Maximizing The Possible." *The Saturday Review,* May 1982, p. 12.

Creagan, Edward T., M.D.: "Psychosocial Issues in Oncologic Practice." *Mayo Clinic Proceedings.*, February 1993, Vol. 68, pp. 161-167.

Dawson, John J.: *The Cancer Patient.* Minneapolis: Augsburg Publishing House, 1978.

Derogatis, Leonard R., Ph.D., Kourlesis, Suzanne M., M.A.: "An Approach to Evaluation of Sexual Problems in the Cancer Patient." *CA-A Cancer Journal for Clinicians,* Vol. 31, No. 1, January/February 1981, pp. 46-50.

DeVita, Vincent T. Jr. M.D.: "The Next Fifteen Years." *The Journal of Cancer Program Management,* August 1986, p. 15.

Diekmann, Judy; Frank-Stromberg, Marilyn; Segalla, Mike; Wright, Penelope S.:"Psychological Impact of the Cancer Diagnosis." *Oncology Nursing Forum,* Vol. 11, No. 3, May/June 1984, pp. 16-22.

Dollinger, Malin, Ernest Rosenbaum and Greg Cable: *Everyone's Guide to Cancer Therapy.* Kansas City: Andrews and McNeel, 1991.

Donnan, Kristin E.: "Cancer: A Medical Update for 1988." *McCall's,* January 1988, pp. 69-75.

Dow, Karen Hassey: "The Enduring Seasons in Survival," *Oncology Nursing Forum,* Vol. 17, No. 4, 1990, pp. 511-516.

Dressler, Lynn G.: "Flow Cytometry - Questions and Answers," ACS Cancer Response System (CRS) No. 3103, July 1991.

Eades, Mary Dan, M.D.: *If It Runs in Your Family: Breast Cancer, Reducing Your Risk.* New York: Bantam Books, 1991.

Eating Hints: Recipes and Tips for Better Nutrition During Cancer Treatment. Bethesda, Maryland. Office of Cancer Communication, National Cancer Institute, 1990.

Elmer-Dewitt, Philip: "Danger in the Speed Trap," *TIME,* October 28, 1991, p. 88.

Ezzell, Carol: "Power Line Static," *Science News,* Vol. 140, September 28, 1991, pp. 203-205.

Facing Forward: A Guide for Cancer Survivors. National Cancer Institute. NIH Publication No. 90-2424, July 1990.

Faulkner, Ann: "Reclaiming a Body Image." *Community Outlook,* May 1985.

Feste, Catherine: *The Physician Within.* Minneapolis: Chronimed Publishing, Revised Edition, 1993.

"Fickle Fields: EMF's and Epidemiology," *Science News,* November 30, 1991, p. 357.

Fiore, Neil A.: *The Road Back to Health*. New York: Bantam Books, 1991.

Friedman, Bonnie Denmark: "Coping with Cancer: A Guide for Health Care Professionals." *Cancer Nursing*, April 1980, pp. 105-110.

Gawain, Shakti: *Creative Visualization*. New York: Bantam Books, 1990.

Granai, Cornelius O. III, M.D., et al: "Female Sexuality and Cancer," *Clinical Advances in Oncology Nursing,* Vol. 3, No. 2, Winter, 1991.

Grier, Sue: "Sexuality and Women with Cancer: Nursing Implications." *Oncology Patient Care*, August 1992, pp. 5-9.

Griffin, James D., M.D.: "Clinical Applications of Colony Stimulating Factors," *Oncology*, January 1988, pp. 15-20.

"High Expectations for Colony Stimulating Factors," *Journal of National Cancer Institute*, Vol. 83, No. 7, April 3, 1991, pp. 470-471.

Immunology and Cancer, American Cancer Society Professional Educational Publication 88-50M-No. 3472-PE, 1988.

Janerich, Dwight T., et al: "Lung Cancer and Exposure to Tobacco Smoke in the Household," *New England Journal of Medicine,* September 6, 1990, pp. 632-636.

Johnson, Judith, R.N., Ph.D.: "The Effects of a Patient Education Course on Persons With a Chronic Illness," *Cancer Nursing,* April 1982, pp. 118-125.

Jones, Sandra Connell, M.A.: "Hospice Care: Emphasizing the Quality of Life, Rather Than the Length," *COPING*, Fall 1992, p. 55.

Kalter, Suzy: *Looking Up: The Complete Guide to Looking Good and Feeling Good for the Recovering Cancer Patient*. New York: McGraw-Hill, 1987.

Kaplan, Mimi: "Viewpoint: The Cancer Patient." *Cancer Nursing*, April 1983, pp. 103-105.

Kauffman, Danette G.: *Surviving Cancer: A Practical Guide For Those Fighting to Win.* Washington, D.C.: Acropolis Books,, 1989.

Kubler-Ross, Elisabeth: *Death: The Final Stage of Growth.* Englewood Cliffs: Prentice-Hall, 1975.

Lamb, Margaret A.: Woods, Nancy F.. "Sexuality and the Cancer Patient." *Cancer Nursing*, April 1981, pp. 137-144.

Langone, J.: "Cancer: Cautious Optimism." *Discover,* March 1986, pp. 41-46.

Larschan, Edward J. with Richard J. Larschan: *The Diagnosis is Cancer.* Palo Alto: Bull Publishing, 1986.

Laurence, Leslie: "Patient, Heal Thyself." *SELF,* October 1991, p. 141.

Lazlo, John, M.D.: *Understanding Cancer.* New York: Harper & Row, 1987.

Lerner, Helene, with Roberta Elins.: *Stress Breakers.* Minneapolis: CompCare Publications, 1985.

Lerner, Irving J., M.D., and B. J. Kennedy, M.D.: "The Prevalence of Questionable Methods of Cancer Treatment in the United States," ACS Publication 92-25M-No. 3022, 1992.

Loeffler, Jay S., M.D., et al: "Radiosurgery for Brain Metastases," *Principles & Practice of Oncology Updates*, Volume 5, Number 2, February 1991, pp.

Mandel, A.: "Hormone Receptors and Breast Cancer," *New England Journal of Medicine*, Vol. 309, 1983, p. 1343.

Meichenbaum, Dr. Donald: *Coping With Stress*. New York: Facts on File, 1983.

Moinpour C., Feigl, P., Metch, B, et al.: "Quality of Life Endpoints in Cancer Clinical Trials," *Journal of National Cancer Institute* 81: 485-495, 1989.

Morra, Marion, and Potts, Eve: *Choices: Realistic Alternatives in Cancer Treatment.* New York: Avon Books, 1987.

Nazario, Sonia L.: "Breast Cancer Researchers Try New Technique," *The Wall Street Journal*, July 31, 1992, p. B-1.

Northouse, Laurel L.: "Living With Cancer." *American Journal of Nursing,* May 1981, pp. 961-962.

Osborne, C. Kent: "DNA Flow Cytometry in Early Breast Cancer: A Step in the Right Direction (Editorial)," *Journal of National Cancer Institute*, Vol. 81, No. 18, September 20, 1989, pp. 1344-1345.

Osoba, David (ed.): *Effect of Cancer on Quality of Life.* Boca Raton, FL: CRC Press, 1991.

"Quality of Life Assessment in Cancer Clinical Trials," *Oncology Bulletin*, March 1993, pp. 14-17.

Questions and Answers About Pain Control. New York: American Cancer Society, 1983.

Radiation Therapy and You: A Guide to Self Help During Treatment. Bethesda, Maryland: Office of Cancer Communication, National Cancer Institute, January 1990.

"Relieving Pain (Parts I and II)," *BMT* Newsletter, March 1993 and May 1993.

Renshaw, Domeena C.: "Sexual and Emotional Needs of Cancer Patients." *Clinical Therapeutics*, Vol. 8, No. 3, 1986, pp. 242-246.

Robinson, Alice M.:"Stress Can Make You—Or Break You." *RN,* November 1975, pp. 73-77.

Rosenbaum, Isadora and Ernest.; Stoklosa, Jean; Bullard, David: *Sexuality and Cancer.* San Francisco: Regional Cancer Foundation (adapted from *Mind and Body: A Rehabilitation Guide for Cancer Patients and Their Families* by Ernest H. Rosenbaum, M.D., and Isadora R. Rosenbaum. Palo Alto: Bull Publishers, 1979.

"Rosenberg, Steven A.: (An Interview)", *OMNI*, August 1993, pp. 71-95.

Runowicz, Carolyn D., M.D.: "Advances in Screening and Treatment of Ovarian Cancer," *CA-A Journal for Cancer Clinicians*, Nov./Dec. 1992, pp. 327-343.

Ryder, Brent (ed.): *The Alpha Book on Cancer and Living*. Alameda, CA: Alpha Institute, 1993.

Ryder, Brent (ed): "Sex and the Cancer Patient." *The Lancet*, February 25, 1984, pp. 432-33.

Sexuality and Cancer: For the Man Who Has Cancer, and His Partner. American Cancer Society Publication 4658-PS, 1988.

Sexuality and Cancer: For the Woman Who Has Cancer, and Her Partner. American Cancer Society Publication 4657-PS, 1988.

Siegel, Mary-Ellen: "What Every Woman Should Know About Ovarian Cancer," *COPING*, January 1991, p. 29.

Simonton, O. Carl; Matthews-Simonton, Stephanie; Creighton, James L.: *Getting Well Again*. New York: Bantam Books, 1978.

Spiegel D., Bloom J., Kraemer H.C., Gottheil E.: "The Effect of Psychosocial Treatment on Survival of Metastatic Breast Cancer Patients: A Randomized Prospective Outcome Study," The *Lancet*, October 14, 1989, pp. 888-891.

"Stereotactic Gamma Knife Radiosurgery," *Association for Brain Tumor Research*, Spring 1989, pp. 3-4.

Stewart, Susan K.: *"Bone Marrow Transplants: A Book of Basics for Patients,"* Highland Park, IL: BMT Newsletter, 1992.

Stewart, Susan K.: *Stress!* Chicago: American Hospital Association, 1977.

Taking Time: Support for People with Cancer and the People Who Care About Them. National Cancer Institute NIH Publication No. 91-2059, December 1990.

Teamwork: The Cancer Patient's Guide to Talking With Your Doctor, National Coalition for Cancer Survivorship (NCCS) Publication No. 5868-1, April 1991.

"Treatment of Early-Stage Breast Cancer," (NIH Consensus *Conference Report),* JAMA, January 16, 1991, Vol. 265, No. 3, pp. 391-395.

"Update: Prostate Cancer Research," *COPING,* Fall 1992, p. 54.

Walbroehl, Gordon S.: "Sexuality in Cancer Patients." *AFP,* January 1985, pp. 153-158.

Weiss, Rick: "Breast Cancer: Every Woman's Worst Fear." *American Health,* September 1992, pp. 49-57.

What Are Clinical Trials All About? U.S. Department of Health and Human Services, National Cancer Institute Pub. No. 90-2706, December 1989.

What You Should Know About Cancer. Duke University Comprehensive Cancer Care Center, 1982.

Index